2/3/16
#22.99

CONCEIVING

PREVENTING AND TREATING INFERTILITY

Pierre Miron M.D., Ph.D.
Mathieu Provençal Ph.D.

CONCEIVING
PREVENTING AND TREATING INFERTILITY

with the collaboration
of Denis Gingras Ph.D.
Foreword by Julie Snyder
Translated by Barbara Sandilands

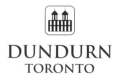

DUNDURN
TORONTO

Copyright © 2015 Les Éditions du Trécarré

Originally published as Concevoir : prévenir et traiter l'infertilité.

Published under arrangement with Groupe Librex Inc., doing business under the name
Éditions du Trécarré, Montréal, QC, Canada

Editor: Michael Melgaard
Design: Laura Boyle
Printer: Marquis
Cover Image: Steffen Thalemann/ Image Bank/ Getty Images

Library and Archives Canada Cataloguing in Publication

Miron, Pierre, 1957-
[Concevoir. English]

Conceiving : preventing and treating infertility / Dr. Pierre
Miron, Mathieu Provençal, and Denis Gingras, PhD ; translated by Barbara Sandilands.

(Your health ; 4)
Translation of: Concevoir, prévenir et traiter l'infertilité.
Includes bibliographical references.
Issued in print and electronic formats.
ISBN 978-1-4597-3007-6 (pbk.).--ISBN 978-1-4597-3008-3 (pdf).--ISBN 978-1-4597-3009-0 (epub)

1. Infertility--Prevention. 2. Infertility--Treatment. 3. Reproductive health. I. Gingras, Denis, 1965-, author II. Provençal, Mathieu, 1979-, author III. Sandilands, Barbara , translator IV. Title. V. Title: Concevoir. English

RC889.M5713 2015   616.6'92   C2015-900597-3
                                             C2015-900598-1

2   3   4   5   19   18   17   16   15

 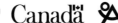 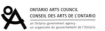

We acknowledge the support of the **Canada Council for the Arts** and the **Ontario Arts Council** for our publishing program. We also acknowledge the financial support of the **Government of Canada** through the **Canada Book Fund** and **Livres Canada Books**, and the **Government of Ontario** through the **Ontario Book Publishing Tax Credit** and the **Ontario Media Development Corporation**.

Care has been taken to trace the ownership of copyright material used in this book. The author and the publisher welcome any information enabling them to rectify any references or credits in subsequent editions.
J. Kirk Howard, President

The publisher is not responsible for websites or their content unless they are owned by the publisher.

Printed and bound in Canada.

Visit us at
Dundurn.com | @dundurnpress | Facebook.com/dundurnpress | Pinterest.com/Dundurnpress

Dundurn
3 Church Street, Suite 500
Toronto, Ontario, Canada
M5E 1M2

To our parents, who gave us life;
To our spouses, who make it more wonderful every day;
And to our children, whom we love so much and through whom it continues.

Table of Contents

Foreword

Not a day goes by without a woman approaching me or writing to tell me about her problem conceiving a child. And, as you will read later on, this is a theme that affects men as much as women.

One in six couples will suffer from infertility at some point. This book meets a real need, for we don't talk enough about this health problem. We don't anticipate this kind of medical complication when we reach adulthood. When we talk about fertility, we're talking about life. Do young women with cancer know that they have the right to freeze their eggs before beginning certain treatments that may make them sterile?

In England, Dr. Robert Edwards, of Cambridge University, and Dr. Patrick Steptoe changed the course of medical history by bringing about the birth of Louise Brown, the first baby created through in vitro fertilization (IVF), on July 25, 1978. Little Louise, known as a test-tube baby, became the embodiment of hope for millions of infertile couples from that day forward.

Since then, thanks to research and technological improvements, five million IVF babies have been born around the world, and Dr. Edwards was awarded the 2010 Nobel Prize for medicine.[1]

In the past, fertility was a taboo subject. People were ashamed of being infertile and suffered in silence. It was a great day when a courageous Céline Dion, the biggest female star on the planet, stated openly that she was expecting a child after undergoing IVF. Louise Brown may be the most famous little girl conceived in vitro, but René-Charles would become the best-known little boy born as a result of this medical technique.

In Germany, Australia, Austria, Belgium, Denmark, Spain, France, Israel, New Zealand,

1. European Society of Human Reproduction and Embryology (ESHRE), "The world's number of IVF and ICSI babies has now reached a calculated total of 5 million," July 1, 2012.

Norway, the Netherlands, and Sweden, IVF treatment and costs have been successfully covered by the government for several years.

In Quebec, since IVF has been made available to everyone, new families are being born, are thriving, and are contributing to the momentum, development, and prosperity of the people of Quebec.

I want to thank the politicians, men and women, of all parties who recognized the need to cover the cost of treatments to cure infertility. I want to stress that I paid for the treatments for my son and daughter myself, at three clinics in Montreal and one in New York. I've fought for the men and women who didn't have the means to cure their disease, well aware that this was not the easiest cause to defend and that I wasn't going to win everyone's sympathy by becoming its standard-bearer.

Some people occasionally call into question the IVF program, saying it costs too much. Yet in our presentations on behalf of the Association des couples infertiles du Québec (Quebec's association for infertile couples) then-president Caroline Amireault's lawyer, Karine Joizil's, and mine, were guided by Dr. Annie Janvier's report, tabled in the National Assembly on March 29, 2006. On behalf of the Society of Neonatologists of Quebec and the Association des pédiatres du Québec, the report requested as a first step that: "The Quebec health system must manage infertility treatment in the same way as treatment for other health problems. Government coverage of infertility treatment would avoid treating some patients differently depending on their financial situation. This would eliminate many conflicts of interest and make it possible to dramatically reduce the rate of multiple pregnancies, neonatal and

pediatric complications, and, as a result, government health care costs."

A pro-natal policy including IVF financing is above all a highly profitable investment for society. A study published in 2008 in the *American Journal of Managed Care* estimates a return on investment from IVF in the order of 700 percent.[2] A society can't go wrong when it invests in having more children.

I'm thrilled that this book has been written. By clearly explaining how to prevent infertility, the steps in investigating it, and its various treatments and drugs, Pierre Miron and his colleagues are finally helping couples to better understand and prepare themselves for the obstacle course that lies ahead.

Last, I wish infertile couples great courage, and my thoughts are with those women who will have to undergo many blood tests, examinations, injections, hormonal roller-coaster rides, treatments, etc. Behind every test-tube baby is a woman who's taken every test available in the hope of becoming a fulfilled mother.

To couples who haven't yet seen results, I'll paraphrase Charles de Gaulle by saying: "You've lost a battle, but you haven't lost the war."

To parents who have longed for a child but been unable to have one, I congratulate you for having done everything you could. You'll be better equipped to grieve and to calmly consider another way of becoming parents.

---

2 M.P. Connolly, MHE, Michael Pollard, Ph.D., Stijn Hoorens, MS.c, Brian Kaplan, MD, Selwyn P. Oskowitz, MD, and Sherman J. Silber, MD, "Long-Term Economic Benefits Attributed to IVF-Conceived Children: A Lifetime Tax Calculation," *American Journal of Managed Care* (2008), study funded by the RAND Corporation of Santa Monica (CA) and Ferring International Center (Switzerland).

When my four-year-old daughter, Romy, born through in vitro fertilization (thank you, Dr. Seang Lin Tan), turns sixteen, I will give her this book so that she will clearly understand that her life choices will influence her ability to have children. And I'll tell her that, in spite of all the ovarian stimulation I underwent, I had only one egg that was able to produce, despite everything, a six-cell embryo of average quality. And that embryo was you, my love. You spent two days outside my body but you'll spend your whole life in my heart.

I will also give it to my big boy, Thomas, now eight, with whom I became pregnant "naturally" between two IVF treatments (thanks to Dr. Miron), for I sincerely hope to be a grandmother one day. My son, you are a gift from God. Your birth changed my life. Because of you, on May 17, 2005, I became another woman, I became a mommy, your mommy forever.

Your daddy cried a lot at both your births and I'm crying again as I write these lines. But they are tears of happiness.

Miracles do exist; my thanks to IVF specialists for giving the good Lord a helping hand.

Julie Snyder
Television Host and Producer

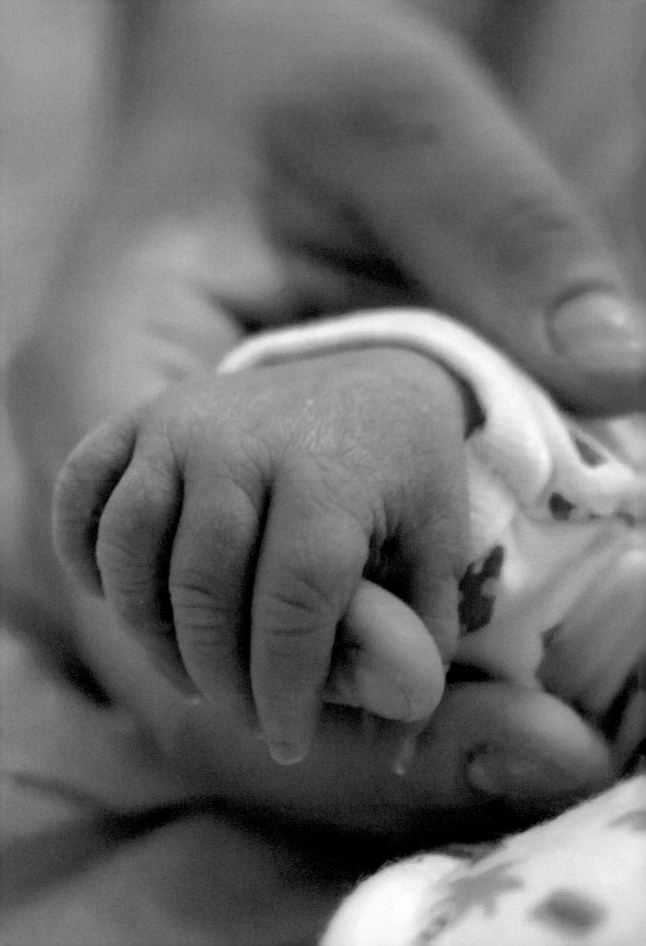

Introduction

A little of us is in the one who leaves and when someone is born a little of all of us becomes someone else.

— GASTON MIRON (1928–1996)

Approximately fifteen thousand generations of human beings have followed each other on Earth since the first members of our species, Homo sapiens, appeared nearly two hundred thousand years ago. Almost all of these people are dead, most of them for a very long time, but they nonetheless live on in us; it is because these billions of individuals were able to survive and reproduce in spite of hostile conditions that human beings have managed to go on century after century and become the most extraordinary animal species to have ever inhabited this planet. We place great importance — and with good cause — on the precious nature of our existence and on the importance of making the most of our brief time on Earth; however, we must not forget that, from a biological standpoint, our lives fit into a much broader context, in which each of us represents a link between the past, bequeathed by our ancestors, and the future of the human species, which will be embodied in our children and their descendants. Every living being must one day die; the only way the human adventure can continue is by adding new links to the great chain of life, ensuring the reproduction of the species before death inevitably occurs. It's through our children that we become immortal.

Yet reproduction is not simply a question of survival, especially today, when contraception means that sexual urges can be dissociated from the conception of children. Nowadays, having children is usually a rational choice, a decision much more tied to emotions than to the survival instinct, and one which is usually weighed carefully so as to integrate the child as harmoniously as possible into family life. This desire for children may take several forms; for some, starting a family is a special way not just to perpetuate the family line, but, even more importantly, to pass on their values and traditions. For others, children are the couple's ultimate accomplishment; they feel the pride (and sometimes the despair!) of discovering in them certain characteristic traits of both parents and of being there, in real time, as they develop through the years. The reasons for wanting a family are many, but they all have in common a couple's desire to see their lives enriched by children, to be amazed by their beauty and the spontaneity of their laughter, or perhaps to be moved by their vulnerability, their innocence, and their unconditional love. Above all, we want children so we can love them and make the most of the great joy this love brings us.

The desire for children can, however, become a cruel disappointment when it runs up against repeated failures to conceive and remains unsatisfied after several months or even several years of trying. Despite society's ever greater openness to everything related to sexuality, infertility paradoxically is still a taboo subject, little understood by the public. Yet up to one couple in six has to deal with an inability to conceive, with the absence of children profoundly upsetting plans for the future and, in some cases, even calling into question the meaning they wanted to give to their lives. Being infertile is a problem that's very hard to accept, for it goes right to the deepest part of ourselves, to that which defines us as human: our ability to give life.

The aim of this book is to inform infertile couples by presenting, as simply as possible, the sum of current knowledge about the causes of infertility and the medical approaches that can be undertaken to

overcome this problem. In recent years, remarkable progress has been made in reproductive medicine, enabling millions of people all over the world to conceive a child despite an infertility problem affecting one or both partners. The impact of these medical advances is particularly significant in certain parts of the world, notably in Quebec, where the government now covers the costs of assisted reproductive procedures, thus giving hope to all infertile couples, irrespective of their income or social status, of realizing their dream of having a child.

While medicine can in many cases treat infertility effectively by facilitating the fertilization of an egg by a sperm, parents also have a major role to play in this process. Creating a child is not just about the fusion of reproductive cells; it's also a matter of creating optimal conditions for those cells to develop in, of doing whatever is necessary so that the embryo can develop as it should, leading to the birth of a healthy child able to live up to its full potential. This means that whether conception occurs naturally or whether medical assistance must be sought to reproduce, all parents have to cope with the same anxieties about the result of a pregnancy, since the excitement caused by the impending arrival of the child is often mixed with fear that something unfortunate will happen that could negatively affect its future.

These concerns are completely legitimate and we believe it's important to face them as directly as possible. To do this, we first have to answer a fundamental question: do we really know how to conceive a child? The question may make us smile, given that sexuality is everywhere in our lives, but do we really know how an egg and a sperm manage to fuse and, all by themselves, develop into a human being made up of many hundreds of billions of cells? Are we aware that this process of fertilization is strongly influenced by a whole range of environmental and lifestyle factors? That the lifestyle habits of the parents, both mother and father, have a key influence on the health of the eventual child, often even before conception? Or indeed that the environment in which the fetus develops will in large part determine its risk of disease in adulthood? What medical resources are available to ensure that the pregnancy proceeds normally and that the child has no abnormalities? It's worth considering these questions, for reproductive biology remains a phenomenon whose extraordinary complexity is still unsuspected by the vast majority of us.

It's in this spirit that we present this overview of the processes involved in conceiving a child and the medical approaches available for treating infertility, as well as the main factors that can affect the development of the fetus. We hope to succeed in sharing with you our amazement at the beauty and complexity of what truly is the great miracle of life.

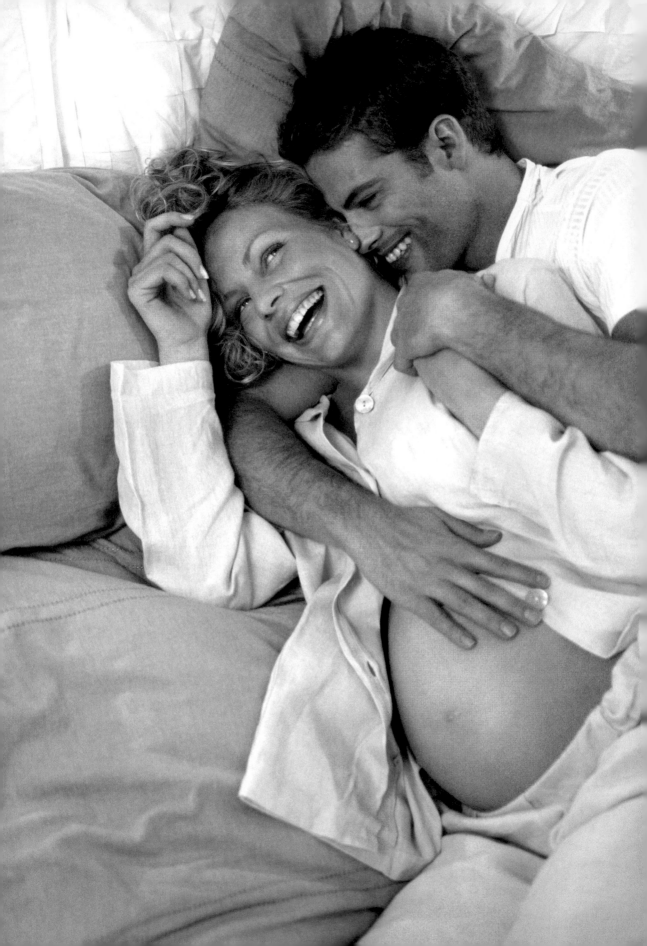

CHAPTER 1

The Benefits of Sex

Love makes us dizzy, but its dizziness, however
intolerable it may be, is an infinite pleasure.
— Hubert Aquin (1929–1977)

"Tell me, Mommy, where do babies come from?" This question, seemingly so simple, actually summarizes all by itself human beings' insatiable curiosity about their origins, as well as our fascination with the mysteries surrounding the conception of a child. What's more, it's thanks to this incessant questioning, probably as old as humanity itself, that we have become the only animals to have understood that there is a direct connection between reproduction and sexuality, a "discovery" that played a major role in the establishment of stable family structures and the emergence of civilizations.

The connection between sexuality and reproduction has long caused parents of curious children many headaches, because of the taboo surrounding everything directly or even remotely related to sex. This embarrassment is clearly illustrated by the impressive number of more or less improbable metaphors that have been invented by most cultures to respond to these legitimate questions; yet swans, bees, or even cabbage leaves are not really adequate to explain the "mysteries of life"! Fortunately, the awkwardness surrounding sexuality is becoming more and more a thing of the past, and society is so open nowadays that we are aware quite early on of the sexual aspects of conceiving a child.

Having a more open mind with respect to sexuality does not, however, mean that we are much better informed about the mechanisms involved in conceiving a child. We often forget this, but sexual relations are just the visible part of an incredibly complex process, whose functioning remains vague for a majority of human beings. Before discussing the factors that can influence reproductive success, we believe it's useful to give a brief overview of the main events that govern the production of female and male reproductive cells and create the conditions that cause them to meet. Better understanding the biology of reproduction is surely the best way to appreciate even more how precious human existence is!

THE REPRODUCTIVE CELLS

Because their physiological functions are so totally different, the female and male reproductive systems represent the main anatomical difference between the two sexes (figure 1).

In women, this system centres on the uterus, the key organ of reproduction, due to its role in fetal development. Its lower portion is connected to the vagina through the cervix, while the upper portion is indirectly linked to the ovaries via the Fallopian tubes. During intercourse, some of the sperm released into the vagina manage to pass through the cervix and the uterine cavity, travel through the Fallopian tubes, and come into contact with an egg released by the ovaries. The fertilized egg then travels to the uterus, where it implants itself in the highly vascularized lining (the endometrium) and begins to develop.

Male reproductive anatomy is simpler, since the function of the testicles is basically to produce sperm cells and send them out through the penis. During ejaculation, sperm temporarily stored in the epididymis, a reservoir next to the testicle, travel through the vas deferens, mix with protective liquids secreted by the seminal vesicles and the prostate, and are excreted in semen.

Just like the man and woman who produce them, the sperm and the egg are very different, yet complementary (figure 2). The most dramatic difference is without doubt that of size: whereas the egg is one of the human body's largest cells (a tenth of a millimetre, or the equivalent of a grain of sand), the sperm cell is one of the smallest, its head measuring only a few thousandths of a millimetre. The sperm's small size is, however, compensated for by its mobility: it's the only cell in the body with a flagellum, a structure that enables it to travel at a relatively high linear speed (from $20\text{--}100^2\text{m/s}$)

ANATOMY OF THE FEMALE AND MALE REPRODUCTIVE SYSTEMS

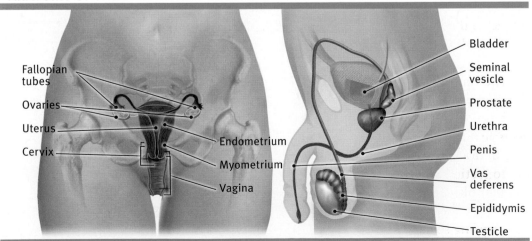

Fallopian tubes
Ovaries
Uterus
Cervix
Endometrium
Myometrium
Vagina

Bladder
Seminal vesicle
Prostate
Urethra
Penis
Vas deferens
Epididymis
Testicle

FIGURE 1

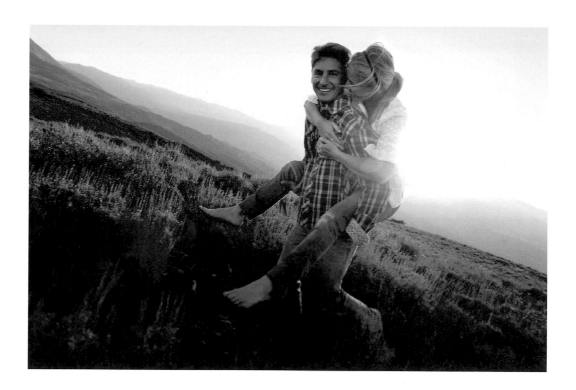

and cover the distance separating it from the egg. These differences illustrate a fundamental characteristic of sexual reproduction: female gametes have to provide the large amount of energy the development of a child requires and are thus bigger and immobile, waiting to be fertilized by male gametes. To do this, the male gametes have to play a much more active role, be very motile and be present in large numbers so that some of them can reach the egg.

The only characteristic the egg and sperm have in common is that they each contain half of the maternal and paternal genetic material. It must be remembered that from a strictly biological point of view, reproduction has an objective in which feelings play absolutely no part: the individual's goal is to pass on his or her genes to offspring so as to ensure the survival of the species. In rudimentary organisms,

such as bacteria, for example, this transmission is very simple: the bacterial cell divides in two, forming two "daughter" cells with exactly the same genes as the "mother" cell. On the other hand, in the vast majority of multicellular living species, reproduction is sexual, involving the fusion of two sets of genetic material, transmitted by a male and a female individual. One of the most significant consequences of this kind of reproduction is to generate a high degree of diversity. The blending of two genetic legacies makes it possible to create new individuals, able to adapt to the world's changing conditions. Hence the great advantage of sex: because of sexual reproduction, children are not only different from their parents; they are, in fact, unique people, the result of a combination of genes that has never existed before and never will again.

EGG AND SPERM: THEY'RE MADE FOR EACH OTHER!

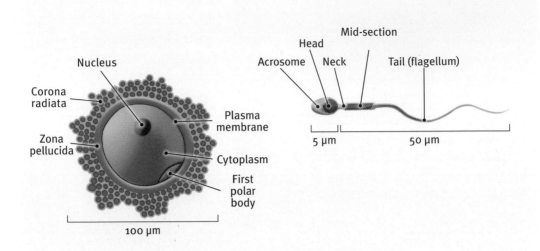

EGG

- The egg is the largest cell in the body (female), roughly 100 μm in length.
- A woman is born with a finite number of eggs (she's really an egg storehouse).
- One egg is released during each menstrual cycle.
- After ovulation, the egg can live for about twenty-four hours.
- The egg can't move around freely. An egg has twenty-three chromosomes — the mother's genetic legacy.
- The egg's twenty-third chromosome is always X.

SPERM

- The sperm cell is the smallest cell in the body (male), about 5 μm long (55 μm with the flagellum).
- After puberty, a man will produce sperm cells every day of his life (he's really a sperm factory).
- Each ejaculate may contain from 20 to 150 million (or more) sperm.
- In ideal conditions, sperm can live up to five days.
- The sperm cell moves around freely using its flagellum: it's the only kind of human cell to have one.
- A sperm has twenty-three chromosomes — the father's genetic legacy.
- The sperm's twenty-third chromosome can be X or Y.

FIGURE 2

22

SEX, A MATTER OF HORMONES

The dramatic changes that occur during puberty are one of the best illustrations of the key role hormones play in reproduction. We often dwell on the external effects of the "hormone surge" that triggers the transition from childhood to adolescence, in both physical development and behaviour, but it's important to realize that these external effects are the visible result of major biochemical changes, whose goal is first and foremost the production of reproductive cells. A crucial step in understanding how a child is conceived, therefore, is to better grasp the major role of hormones in managing this process.

Hormones are chemical messengers, secreted by certain specialized glands, which influence the functioning of organs located in another part of the organism. Somewhat like a thermostat, hormones can self-regulate, adjusting their own production depending on the intensity of the response they cause (figure 3).

For example, if you set a thermostat at a given temperature, it sends an electric signal to activate the heating system and turn on the heat. Once the room temperature reaches the setting on the thermostat, the appliance registers the information and quits sending signals so that the system will stop and not exceed the desired temperature. All the hormone systems in our bodies work in this same way: after they are produced by a gland, hormones are transported in the bloodstream to a target organ where they cause a specific physiological response (building proteins, transporting sugar, producing other hormones, etc.). The intensity of this response is in turn recorded by the gland, which, like a

SELF-REGULATION OF HORMONAL SYSTEMS BY FEEDBACK INHIBITION

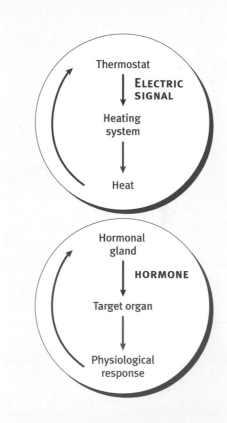

Similar to a thermostat that shuts off when the temperature reaches a certain level, the activity of hormone-producing glands is controlled by the intensity of the physiological response a hormone causes. When this response reaches a specific threshold, a feedback inhibition mechanism is activated (red arrow), stopping hormone secretion.

FIGURE 3

Children Are One of a Kind

Each of our cells has in its nucleus 23 pairs of chromosomes, formed by the combination of a maternal and a paternal chromosome. To reproduce, however, 46 chromosomes from a man cannot simply be joined with 46 chromosomes from a woman: the resulting 92 chromosomes would create a non-viable organism.

The primary function of egg and sperm cells is thus to produce a light version of this genetic material, to cut the number of chromosomes in half by choosing at random one of the two members of each pair. In other words, the parents' genetic heritage is not reproduced as is; a child does not have the same chromosomes as its father or mother, but actually a mixture of the two, in addition to which new combinations of chromosomes are often created when reproductive cells are formed.

---

thermostat, reduces its hormone production to keep the system from getting out of control. This phase of hormonal activity, called feedback inhibition, is extremely important for the entire functioning of the organism, as it allows the various organs to react very quickly to any physiological fluctuation and to re-establish equilibrium by increasing or decreasing hormone production.

The hormonal control of reproduction is based on the same principle in both men and women. In both cases, however, the situation is slightly more complex, since the control centre (the "thermostat") is located in the hypothalamus, a small region of the brain whose role is to integrate all the pieces of information that are received from the outside and relayed to the brain by the nervous system. The hypothalamus is not itself a hormonal gland, however, and cannot manage all of the systems that depend on hormone secretion on its own; to do so, it must rely on the collaboration of the pituitary gland, located nearby, which specializes in producing hormones whose role is to regulate a number of physiological processes, including reproduction.

In concrete terms, this partnership is made possible by certain specialized neurons that release a neurohormone called gonadotropin-releasing hormone (GnRH), which in turn stimulates the pituitary to produce a class of hormones called gonadotropins (FSH and LH) in response (see box, page 25). These hormones then travel to the reproductive organs (ovaries or testicles) where they stimulate the development of the sex hormones required for reproductive cells to mature (figure 4). In women, estrogen controls the menstrual cycle, causing ovulation, while in men testosterone acts locally to cause sperm cells to mature. In both cases, levels of these hormones are continually monitored by the hypothalamus and the pituitary gland so as to constantly adjust production by increasing or decreasing, according to need, the amounts of GnRH, FSH, and LH secreted. The hormonal axes that connect the hypothalamus, the pituitary, and the gonads (ovaries or testicles) are therefore the cornerstone of sexuality, a highly efficient system on which reproductive success rests. Sex really is all about hormones!

Star Hormones

The maturation of eggs and sperm relies on the same hierarchy of hormones that connect the brain to the female and male reproductive systems. Among the many hormones involved, three play a particularly important role.

GnRH: Gonadotropin-releasing hormone (GnRH), also called luteinizing-releasing hormone (LHRH), is reproduction's hormone-in-chief, the one that controls all the events that ultimately lead to the production of reproductive cells. The key role of GnRH derives from its ability to trigger the release of the gonadotropins FSH and LH by the pituitary gland; these two hormones are essential for the production of sex hormones by the gonads. One characteristic of GnRH is its cyclic secretion, in the form of pulses, whose frequency determines which gonadotropins the pituitary will produce in the greatest amounts. While these pulses are relatively regular (every two hours approximately) in men, they vary considerably in the course of the menstrual cycle in women, making the coordination of egg maturation and release by the ovaries possible.

FSH: As its name indicates, the primary function of follicle-stimulating hormone (FSH) is to support the development of the ovarian follicles involved in egg maturation. When FSH secreted by the pituitary gland causes a follicle to reach about 10 millimetres in size, the follicular cells secrete large amounts of estrogen needed for the menstrual cycle to continue. At the same time, the estrogen exerts an inhibiting action on the hypothalamus, which decreases GnRH production, leading to reduced secretion of FSH by the pituitary. This negative feedback control mechanism is important, since reduced levels of FSH prevent smaller follicles from developing. A dominant follicle can then be selected and only one egg will mature.

In men, FSH acts on the Sertoli cells in the walls of the testicles' seminal tubes to support the sperm cell maturation process. FSH stimulates the division of spermatocytes (immature sperm cells) and sensitizes the Sertoli cells to the testosterone produced by the Leydig cells, two processes that play a critical role in sperm cell production.

LH: The secretion of luteinizing hormone (LH) by the pituitary plays an essential role in ovulation. LH also triggers the production of androgens by the follicles, with these hormones acting as precursors to estrogen synthesis. This androgenic function is especially visible in men, in whom the stimulation of Leydig cells by LH is responsible for the production of 95% of the body's testosterone. In addition to its many effects on a whole range of physiological processes, testosterone is absolutely essential for sperm cell maturation, and any imbalance in the levels of this hormone can affect the process.

The brain's participation in controlling sex hormone production also means that external events can influence the hypothalamic-pituitary complex, and thus sexual cycles. This influence is especially conspicuous in women, as a number of environmental factors (chronic stress, powerful emotions, dietary imbalances) can cause changes in the menstrual cycle.

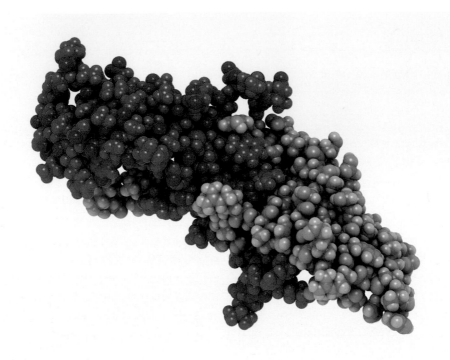

↗ Follicle-stimulating hormone (FSH).

MALE AND FEMALE HYPOTHALAMIC-PITUITARY- GONADAL AXES

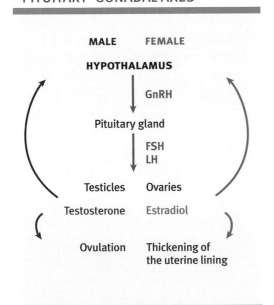

FIGURE 4

THE MENSTRUAL CYCLE

The menstrual cycle is one of the best illustrations of the complexity of the hormonal mechanisms at work in controlling reproduction. The cycle is repeated approximately 450 times from puberty to menopause and is truly an example of physiological "choreography," a perfectly managed performance during which a series of hormones appear one after another in a well-established order to regulate the maturation and expulsion of an egg and create favourable conditions for it to implant in the uterus.

The implementation of such a rigid hormonal control system is necessary since pregnancy is a process that takes a huge amount of energy; the brain's control of hormone production thus ensures that the conditions prevailing inside the body are compatible with the development of an embryo. For example, major imbalances in metabolism (anorexia, morbid obesity, over-training) are interpreted by the hypothalamus as threats to the body's integrity that may interfere with fetal development. In such situations, it's therefore common for GnRH secretion to be disrupted, and for ovulation not to occur. What's more, a feature of the female reproductive system is that all eggs are produced during the female's fetal period, before birth; they remain in a latent state for many years before being used to conceive a child. The role of hormones is to "wake up" these immature eggs, and to stimulate them so they develop and become available for fertilization.

We must therefore remember that the sole goal of the sequence of hormonal events involved in the menstrual cycle is to bring an egg to maturity, to expel it from the ovary so it can meet up with a sperm cell, and to create favourable conditions for an embryo to implant and grow. Each of the three main stages involved is regulated by a specific hormone combination that makes the precise orchestration of the progression of the cycle possible (figure 5).

Follicular Phase
The immature eggs produced during fetal development are stored inside follicles, clusters of cells surrounding the egg whose role is to supply the nutrients and hormones required for it to mature (see page 29). The first phase of the menstrual cycle thus involves stimulating these follicles and encouraging them to develop enough to support the final stages of egg maturation and its release from the ovary.

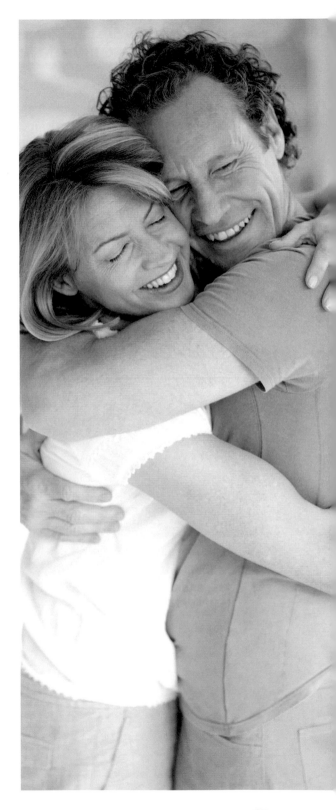

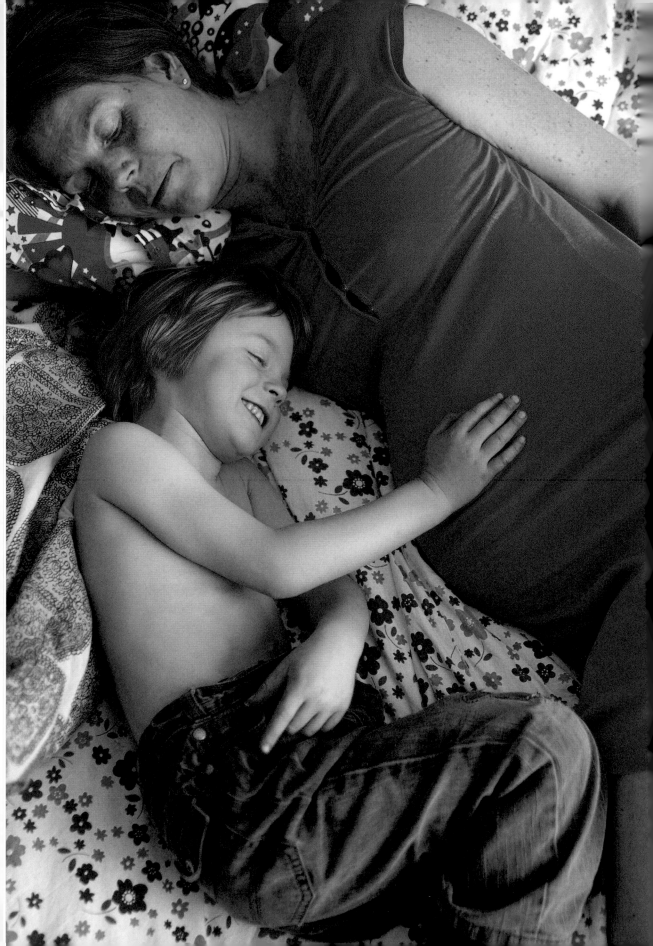

sperm as possible to enhance the likelihood that one of them will succeed in getting past the obstacles between it and the
egg. This dynamic can in a way be compared to the likelihood of reaching a target
a good distance away: statistically speaking, the more missiles you use, the better
the chances that one will reach the target!
And the number of these missiles is impressive: whereas women are born with their
entire egg supply and only approximately
450 will reach maturity between puberty
and menopause, the testicles produce more
than 100 million sperm each day (1,500 per
second), starting at puberty. An eighty-year-
old man will therefore have produced more
than 2,000 billion sperm!

The amazing efficiency of the sperm
production process is due to the seminiferous tubules, a series of compact structures that look somewhat like noodles and
take up most of the space in the testicles.
These seminiferous tubules are separated
from each other by highly vascularized
conjunctive tissue containing the Leydig
cells, whose main role is to produce testosterone in response to the LH secreted
by the pituitary gland.

The testosterone produced next to the
seminiferous tubules plays a crucial role in
sperm maturation (figure 7). The lining of
each tubule is made up of a layer of stem
cells (spermatogonia) and Sertoli cells,
whose role is to nourish the stem cells and
support their differentiation into mature
sperm. After puberty, the stimulation of Sertoli cells by FSH and the production of testosterone by the Leydig cells activate the
spermatogonia, causing them to undergo a
series of changes that will result in the formation of the acrosome, a vesicle (sac) containing enzymes essential for penetrating the

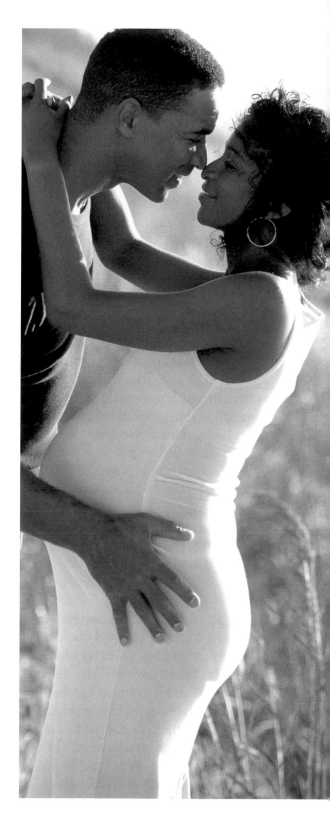

FERTILIZATION

Fertilization is the culmination of all of the hormonal and physiological processes involved in the production and maturation of reproductive cells, and also the most complex. The union of a sperm and an egg does not happen by accident; it's the result of a series of molecular interactions in which the sperm is "sucked" toward the egg, digesting its external membrane so it can pass on the genetic material contained in its head. In concrete terms, sperm that are located near the egg must first make their way through the follicular cells surrounding it (corona radiata) to reach the zona pellucida, a layer where those sperm with an intact plasma membrane and belonging to the same species are selected (this is why sperm from one species cannot fertilize eggs from another). At this stage, receptors on the sperm's surface combine physically with certain proteins in the egg's membrane to anchor them firmly together, marking the beginning of the acrosome reaction.

This is a key moment in fertilization: the acrosome on the sperm's head releases enzymes that break down the zona pellucida and enable the sperm to fuse its membrane with that of the egg in order to transfer the contents of its nucleus. And that's it! But before incorporating the sperm's genetic material, the egg must ensure that more sperm will not penetrate it: as soon as fusion with a sperm has taken place, a series of biochemical events causes an almost instantaneous change (a few milliseconds) in the structure of the pellucid membrane, which lifts up and becomes unstuck from the egg, thus eliminating any possibility of fusion with another sperm (cortical reaction). This protection mechanism means that an egg is always fertilized by a single sperm, preventing the creation of embryos containing superfluous copies of chromosomes, which would not be viable (polyspermia).

To sum up, the fertilization of an egg by a sperm is the result of a series of events carefully staged by the hormonal fluctuations that accompany the menstrual cycle. Despite its complexity, the entire process is astonishingly efficient and fast (figure 9): following ovulation caused by an increase in LH on about the thirteenth day of the cycle, the egg is fertilized in the Fallopian tube during the next twelve to twenty-four hours and begins immediately to migrate to the uterus, which is ready to receive it owing to the changes brought about by progesterone secreted by the corpus luteum. During this migration, the embryo begins to divide, reaching the morula stage (sixteen cells) within two to four days, and then the blastocyst stage, containing a few hundred cells. Barely a week after ovulation, the hatching blastocyst is already implanted in the uterine lining, where it will develop over the next thrity-five to forty weeks, nourished by the placenta, which brings it oxygen and essential nutrients in the mother's blood.

In spite of its beauty and elegance, fertilization remains an extremely delicate process. All of the many hormonal and anatomical factors involved, from the production of the sperm and the egg, to the creation of conditions required for them to make contact and the implantation and growth of the fetus in the uterus, means that the malfunctioning of even one of these stages can upset the whole process and prevent couples from conceiving a child.

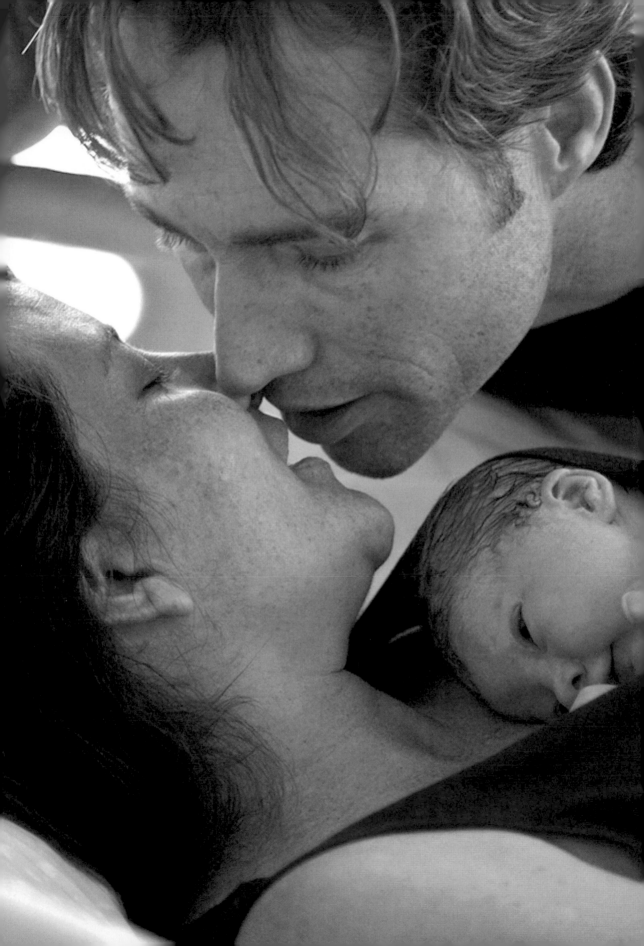

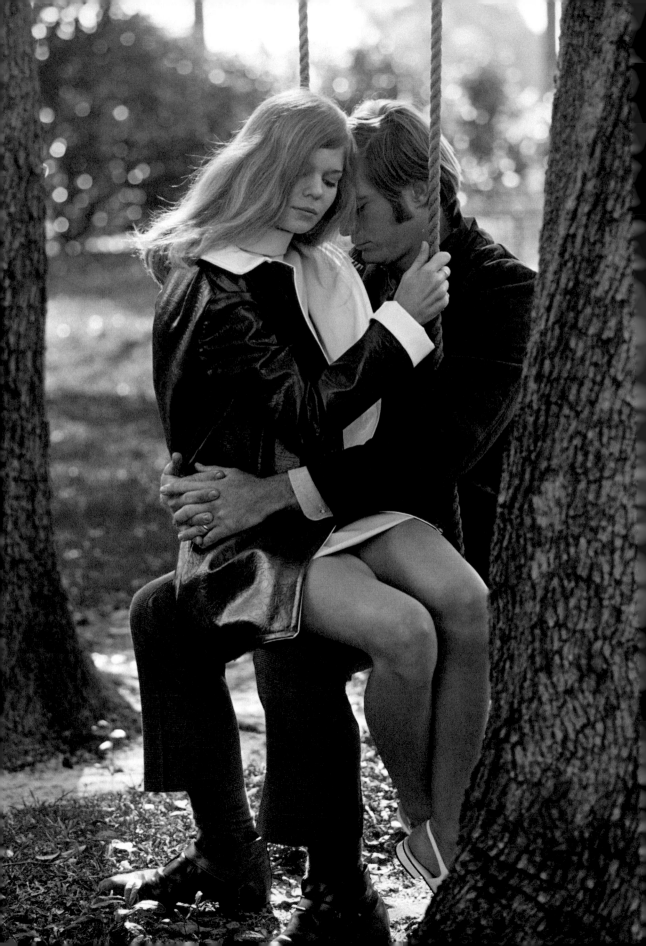

CHAPTER 2

Conception Difficulties

On the straw of this simple bed, the sleep of the little ones, like fresh air and sunshine, will make them more beautiful, brighter, stronger.
— CHARLES-NÉRÉE BEAUCHEMIN (1850–1931)

Few developments have had such a huge impact on the structure and functioning of modern societies as birth control. By dissociating sexuality and reproduction, contraception gave couples, and particularly women, the ability to reconcile their personal and professional lives, making it possible for them to postpone starting a family for a few years, and giving them time to go through the stages necessary for them to achieve their goals and dreams. Whether this means getting a higher education, leading to professions that were formerly almost inaccessible (medicine, engineering, management, etc.), exploring the world through travel, or simply wanting to fully experience a variety of romantic relationships, all these changes have completely redefined the traditional female role and opened up new horizons for women to take their place in society. The desire for children is still there, but over time it has become a more rational choice, depending not just on the emotional and romantic context, but also on when the time feels right to go ahead.

However, being able to control one's fertility while enjoying a regular sex life may give the impression that the opposite is also true — that stopping contraception leads almost automatically to conceiving a child. Yet, this feeling of control over reproductive functions is not always justified: a significant number of couples who have carefully planned the time to start a family and are impatiently awaiting the arrival of a child find themselves dealing with unexpected delays in getting pregnant, unable to conceive or experiencing repeated miscarriages. This is difficult to deal with, not only because the desire for a child remains unfulfilled in the short term, but, even more worrying, because these repeated failures give rise to doubts as to the couple's

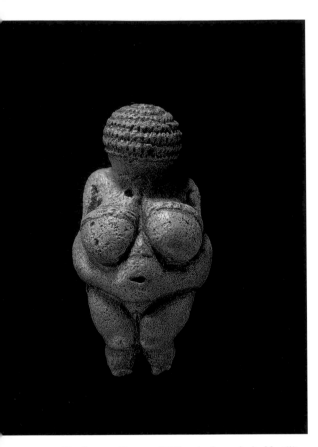

↗ The famous Venus of Willendorf, symbol of fertility.

is, its prevalence in modern societies, and the main factors known to contribute to the decrease in fertility. For as with all essential physiological processes, the success of fertilization can be influenced by a whole range of environmental and sociocultural factors.

HUMAN FERTILITY

The human species is relatively infertile: our fecundability, or the likelihood of conception in each menstrual cycle, is about 25 percent, a much lower percentage than in all other animal species. Part of this difference is due to lower sperm production in men, up to five times less than some animals (figure 10), as well as to a very large proportion of these reproductive cells having abnormal morphological characteristics.

Another factor contributing to lower fertility is the large proportion of human pregnancies that are not carried to term. Nearly a third of embryos that implant themselves in the uterus are expelled before the tenth week of pregnancy, with the vast majority of these miscarriages being caused by non-hereditary chromosomal errors. Pregnancy loss is more common in women under eighteen as well as in those over thirty-five, and its frequency increases with the number of previous children (figure 11). For example, the risk of miscarriage between the sixth and twelfth weeks of pregnancy is from 9 to 12 percent in women under 35 and 50 percent in those forty and over. In 50 to 60 percent of cases, miscarriages are associated with chromosomal abnormalities, mainly trisomies, and thus are indicative of major genetic defects that prevent

fertility and the possibility of achieving this dream in the longer term. Faced with a situation like this, what can couples do? What is a normal time frame for conceiving? Is there anything concrete they can do to enhance their chances of success? And when nothing seems to work, when should they begin to be concerned and see a doctor?

It's important to answer these questions, as infertility disorders are a more widespread problem than we think, and whose causes society knows very little about. Before beginning to examine in detail the medical factors involved in female and male infertility, we believe it's useful to provide a brief overview of what infertility

the development of a viable child. In certain rarer cases, pregnancy loss occurs repeatedly (two miscarriages or more), and this phenomenon can be a significant obstacle to the conception of a child (see page 44).

INFERTILITY

Infertility is generally defined as the inability of a couple to conceive a child after one year of frequent sexual relations without using contraceptives. According to World Health Organization statistics, it is estimated that eighty million people suffer from infertility or subfertility in one form or another, with the problem being especially common in western countries. In Canada, for example, from 10 to 15 percent

of couples are infertile, and this disorder seems to have been steadily on the rise in recent decades. Thus, whereas in 1984 the percentage of couples estimated to have fertility problems was 5 percent, this number had risen to 8.5 percent by 1992, and has reached 15 percent today.

Contrary to what many people think, this decline in fertility is not a strictly female phenomenon: worldwide, the scientific community estimates that ovulatory dysfunction and problems originating in the pelvis (tubal blockage, endometriosis, etc.) are responsible for about 45 percent of cases of infertility, a proportion similar to that caused by factors originating in males (figure 13). In addition, a significant proportion of infertility cases (10 percent) remains unexplained, but is likely due to male and female factors equally.

COMPARISON OF SPERM COUNTS IN VARIOUS MAMMALS

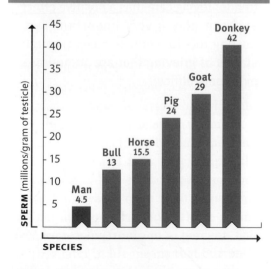

FIGURE 10   Source: Adapted from França et al. in Martinez-Garcia and Regadera (Eds.), 1998.

PROBABILITY OF PREGNANCY LOSS BY MATERNAL AGE

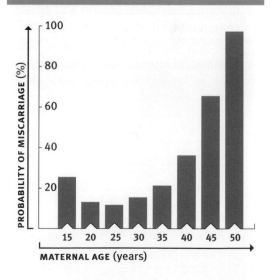

FIGURE 11

contrast to men, who constantly renew their supply of reproductive cells after puberty, the sum total of eggs is created very early on, well before birth (Chapter 1, page 22). A maximum of six to seven million eggs is reached at around twenty weeks' gestation, only one to two million are still there at birth, and their number continues to decrease over time. For example, the ovarian reserve of a thirty-year-old woman only contains 12 percent of the eggs she started out with and only 3 percent by age forty (figure 16). On the other hand, since the number of eggs remaining would, in theory, be sufficient for fertilization to occur, it's probable that the decline in fertility associated with aging might also be attributable to changes in the follicle maturation process during the menstrual cycle and the production of lower quality eggs.

Whatever the reason, while the rate of infertility in women under 30 is less than 10 percent, it rises to 15 percent in the early thirties and 22 percent between 35 and 40. After 40, it's estimated that roughly a third of women cannot get pregnant by natural means (figure 18).

Although male infertility is much less affected by age, it's nonetheless a fact that levels of testosterone decrease by about 1 percent a year after age thirty, with harmful consequences for sperm production. A number of recent observations indicate that the quality of sperm declines significantly with age, especially with regard to the integrity of their genetic material, which increases the risk of infertility, as well as that of transmitting certain abnormalities to the child. For example, the sperm of men forty and over can contain three times as many mutations in their DNA as those of men aged twenty, and recent studies indicate that these mutations are associated with a heightened risk for certain neurological problems, such as schizophrenia or autism spectrum disorders (figure 17).

PERCENTAGE OF CHILDREN BORN TO MOTHERS OVER 30 IN CANADA, 1974–2008

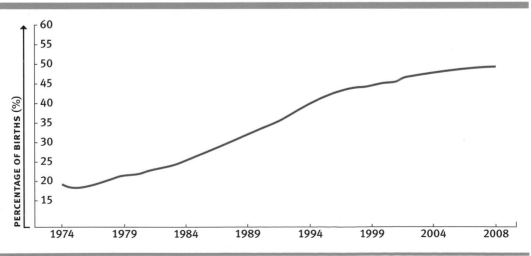

FIGURE 14

Source: Statistics Canada, 2011.

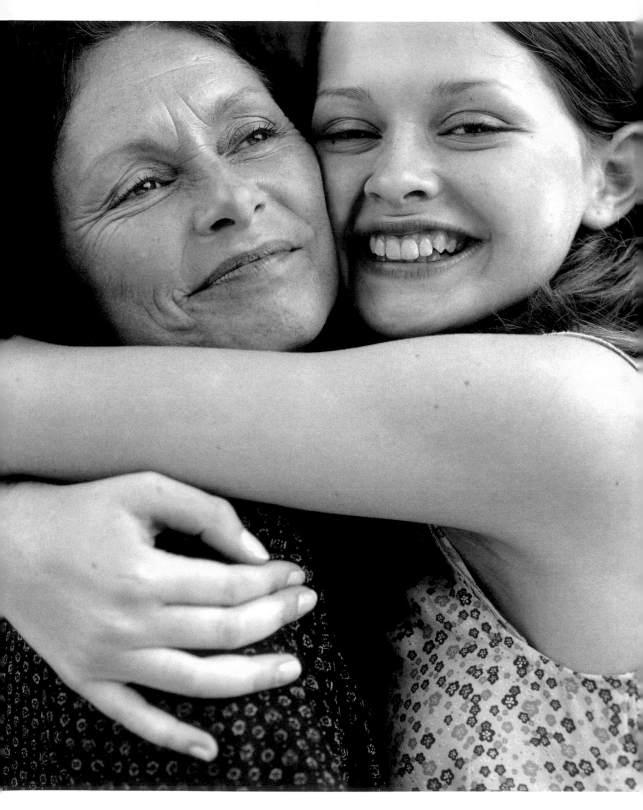

PROBABILITY OF CONCEPTION EACH MONTH BY MATERNAL AGE

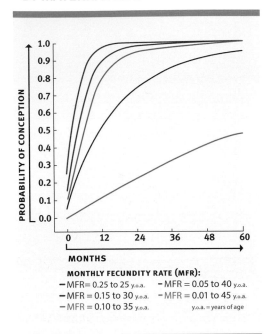

MONTHLY FECUNDITY RATE (MFR):
- MFR= 0.25 to 25 y.o.a.
- MFR = 0.15 to 30 y.o.a.
- MFR = 0.10 to 35 y.o.a.
- MFR = 0.05 to 40 y.o.a.
- MFR = 0.01 to 45 y.o.a.

y.o.a. = years of age

FIGURE 15   Source: Adapted from the NHS (United Kingdom), 2012.

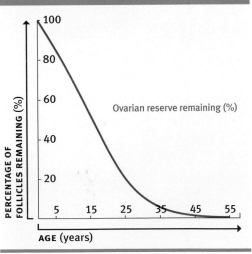

THE ENVIRONMENT

One of the great paradoxes of modern industrialized societies is the major environmental deterioration that has accompanied improvements in people's standard of living. While we have the good fortune to benefit from unprecedented comfort and quality of life, air pollution, global warming, and the countless toxic chemical compounds that contaminate our water and soil are there to remind us that this progress has often come at the cost of damaging the world we live in, and that this situation is likely to cause serious health problems for human beings.

As well as being harmful to health in general, exposure to chemical products can interfere with human reproduction;

DECREASE IN THE OVARIAN RESERVE BY AGE

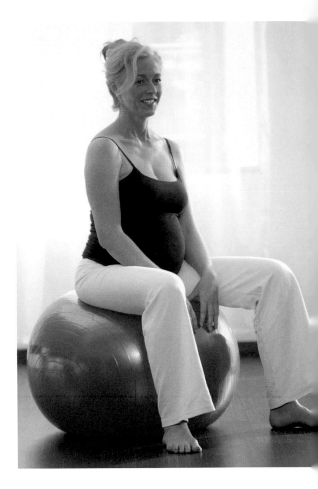

Ovarian reserve remaining (%)

FIGURE 16   Source: Adapted from Wallace et al., 2010.

for example, more than two thousand years ago the Romans noticed that exposure to lead was associated with an increased risk of miscarriage and infertility. Could "modern" environmental aggressors have a similar effect, which would explain the decline in fertility observed during the past century? This question requires an urgent answer, since a large number of chemical compounds in the environment are known to have carcinogenic, mutagenic, and reprotoxic effects, and it's likely this list will get longer, given that as many as one hundred thousand of these compounds have not been tested to date.

In the same vein, a number of studies have reported a significant decline in the quantity of sperm in men in certain parts of the world. For example, a French team has recently revealed that the average concentration of sperm in men aged 18 to 70 has dropped about 33 percent during the past fifteen years, a decrease of approximately 2 percent a year (figure 19). Similar decreases have also been noted in Canada, Belgium, and Scotland, whereas studies done in Finland, as well as in a number of American cities, have not shown major changes in semen quality. These differences suggest that environmental factors capable of damaging male fertility are more likely local in origin.

It's believed that one of these factors could be a group of compounds called "endocrine disruptors." As their name indicates, these molecules are able to interfere with the normal functioning of the hormone system and thus cause undesirable effects in an organism or its offspring. Where reproductive functions are concerned, bisphenol A (BPA), phthalates, and glycol ethers have attracted the most attention to date, as these molecules, found

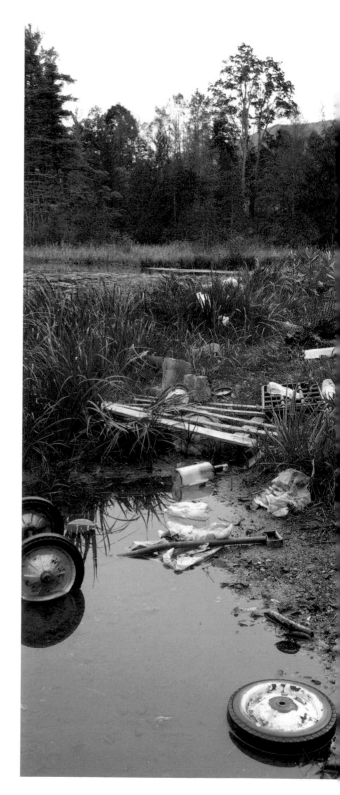

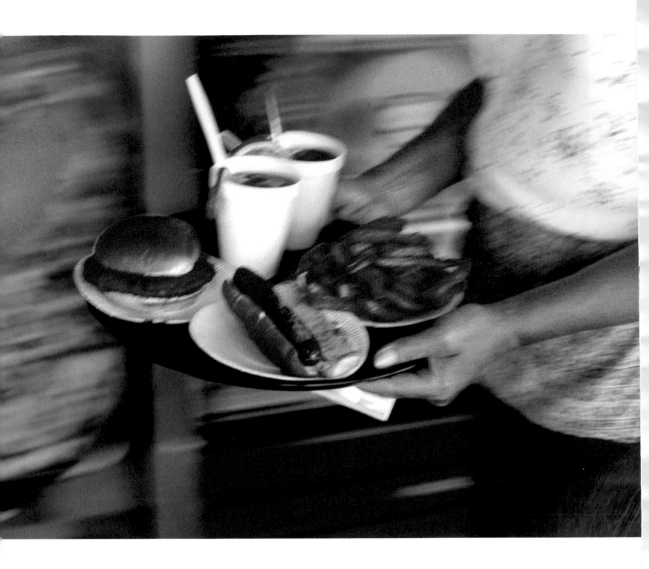

rather ironic that throughout history fertility goddesses — like the Venus of Willendorf — have been depicted as stout women!

Obese women are also at high risk of developing insulin resistance, resulting in the development of type 2 diabetes and, ultimately, metabolic syndrome (a combination of high blood pressure, hyperlipidemia, and diabetes). These metabolic and hormonal imbalances create inflammatory conditions that disrupt ovarian function and cause oligomenorrhea (irregular menstruation) or even amenorrhea (the absence of menstrual periods) if the glycemia is not appropriately treated.

The risk of infertility associated with being overweight does not, however, mean that women having difficulties conceiving have to try to become as thin as possible! Too low a body weight (BMI < 19) is also associated with ovulatory dysfunction (caused by deficiencies of FSH and LH), which considerably increases the risk of infertility. Maintaining a normal weight, with a BMI in the range of 23 to 25, is thus a much more reasonable (and realistic) goal, in addition to which this kind of healthy weight is also linked to a lower risk for all chronic diseases in the population as a whole.

Just as in women, being overweight is also a significant infertility factor in men. The enzyme that turns testosterone into estrogen (aromatase) is more active in the fat cells of obese men; the increase in estrogen that occurs as a result has an inhibiting effect on the hypothalamic-pituitary-testicular axis, diminishes testosterone production, and suppresses spermatogenesis (Chapter 1, page 34). The harmful effect of obesity on fertility can be even greater in cases of type 2 diabetes, since the damage caused to blood vessels by hyperglycemia increases the risk of erectile dysfunction and retrograde ejaculation. This is why recent studies suggest that returning blood sugar to normal levels using insulin-sensitizing agents, such as metformin, might improve semen quality in obese subjects.

The Type of Diet
Aside from the influence of body weight, the precise role of various components of diet in relation to fertility remains poorly understood, but appears to be significant. In women, we know for example that drinking too much coffee (five or more cups a day) is associated with a 50 percent reduction in fertility; lowering daily caffeine intake to less than 250 mg (one or two cups of coffee) is therefore recommended. A study carried out in women aged 20 to 45 showed that those who adopted a Mediterranean-style diet, typically including a generous intake of fruits, vegetables, fish, and whole grains, were approximately 50

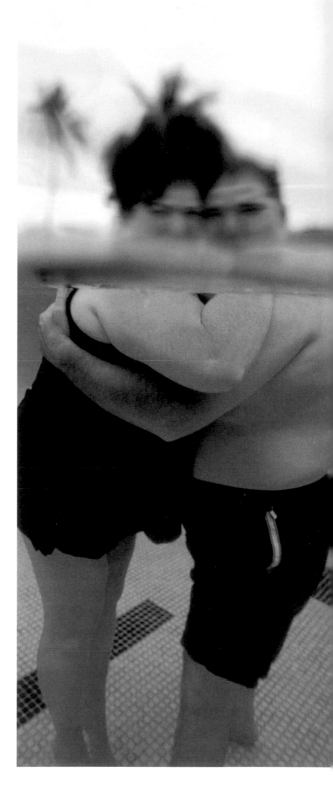

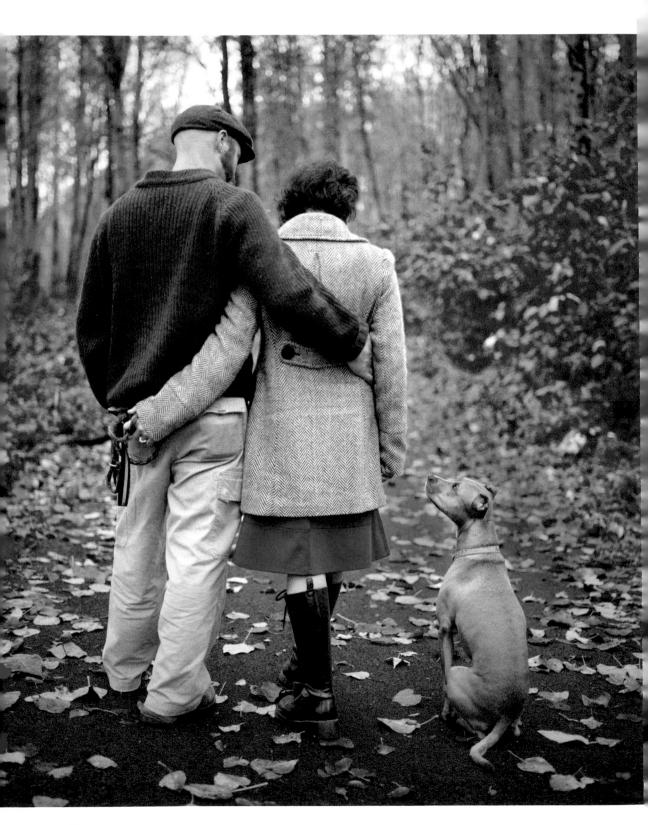

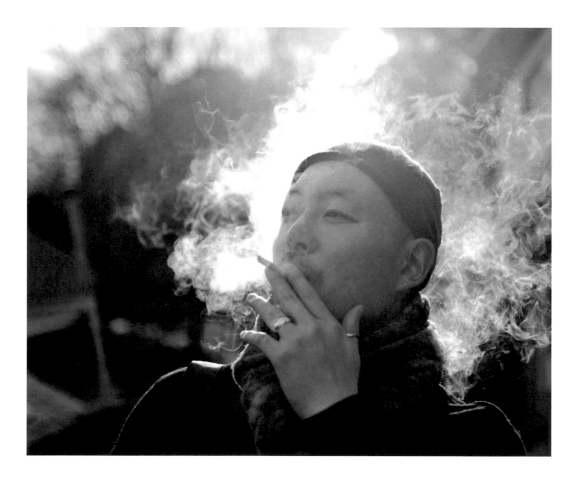

TOBACCO AND OTHER PSYCHOACTIVE SUBSTANCES

While especially known for its disastrous impact on the risk of lung cancer and heart disease, smoking is also the main lifestyle factor associated with the disruption of reproductive function. Nicotine, tar, and the thousands of chemical compounds in cigarette smoke have many harmful effects on the functioning of the female reproductive system: increased risk of ectopic pregnancy, more rapid disappearance of ovarian follicles (atresia), degeneration of the zona pellucida surrounding the eggs, a decline in the quality of the uterine lining that receives the embryo, a drop in estrogen levels, deterioration of the egg's genetic material, etc. As a result, smoking is associated with earlier menopause (on average from one to four years earlier than in non-smokers), more frequent pregnancy losses, and a dramatic increase (60 percent) in the risk of infertility; women who smoke and who begin an assisted reproductive procedure have success rates significantly lower than non-smoking women. For women who smoke and have difficulty conceiving a child, quitting smoking is an essential step toward improving their chances.

The negative impact of tobacco on the male reproductive system is just as significant. Smokers generally have fewer sperm (oligozoospermia) than those

59

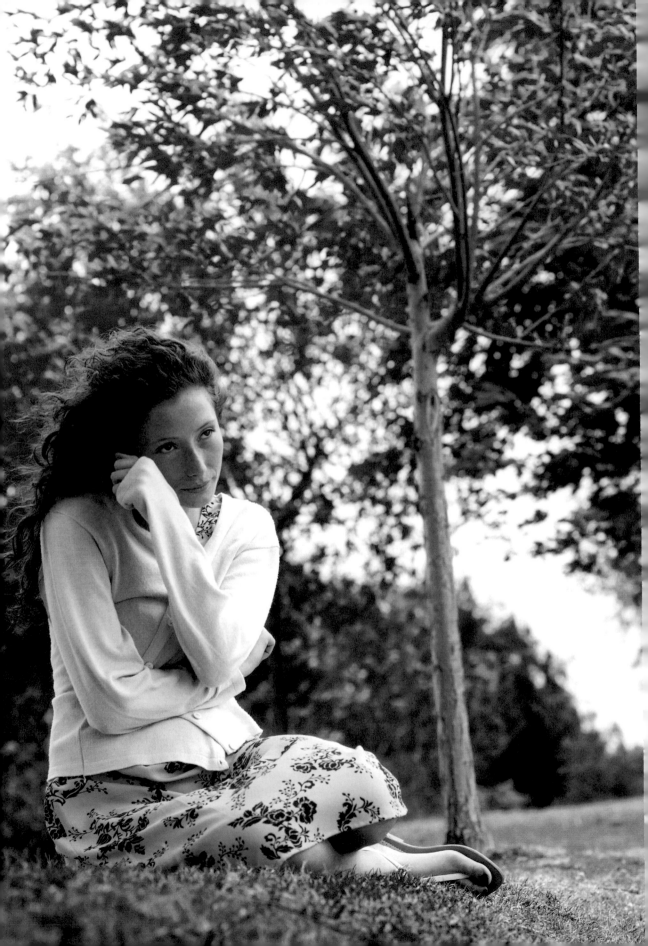

CHAPTER 3

Female Infertility

I walk beside a joy
Beside a joy that is not mine
A joy of mine which I cannot take
— HECTOR DE SAINT-DENYS GARNEAU (1912–1943)[3]

In the past, any failure to conceive was immediately blamed on a problem with female physiology. No excuse was needed to lay the blame for sterility on the woman; it was because her womb was too moist or too hot and let the semen run out or "smothered" it, it was divine punishment for a faith in God that wasn't strong enough, or it was some kind of anatomical defect. Lack of understanding of a woman's internal anatomy certainly did not help develop a more rational view: for example, it was long thought that the uterus was directly connected to the digestive system, which meant that a diagnosis of infertility could be reached simply by placing a garlic clove in the vagina. If the garlic odour could be detected in the woman's breath, she was fertile! Even worse, being infertile branded a woman as an inferior being, unable to fulfil the role nature intended for her. Fortunately, the situation

has improved in many parts of the world, but it's not unusual even today for women to bear the bulk of the burden of infertility, with the psychological consequences and feelings of guilt that are so much a part of being unable to reproduce.

We must however take an optimistic view of the future: female infertility is a medical problem that is gradually becoming better understood and can in many cases be overcome, thanks to the considerable progress made by modern reproductive medicine.

INVESTIGATING FEMALE INFERTILITY

Beginning the fertility evaluation process can be an unsettling experience, both because of anxiety about the diagnosis and the fear of having to undergo various, sometimes painful, procedures. While

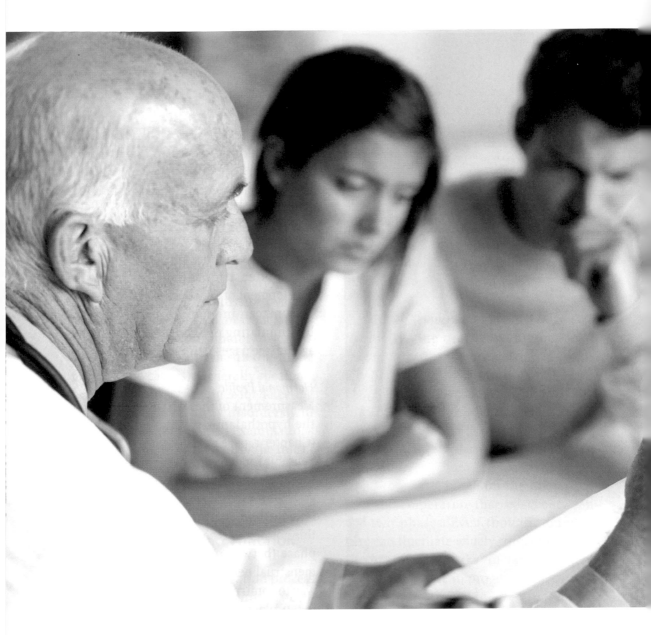

and sex steroid (estrogens, androgens), lactogenic (prolactin), and thyroid hormones, we can, in many cases, find out exactly why ovulation does not occur and what the therapeutic options are for correcting this problem. Anti-Müllerian hormone (AMH), mainly found in the small follicles (pre-antral or early pre-antral), may sometimes be measured to estimate how many good quality eggs there are (ovarian reserve) and to predict how the ovaries will respond to ovulation-inducing agents. Finally, sometimes measuring the levels of other hormones, such as testosterone, 17-hydroxyprogesterone and adrenal DHEAS, also helps determine the exact cause of anovulation with greater accuracy.

Ultrasound

Using transvaginal ultrasound, ovarian volume (approximately 6.5 ml) can be measured and the size and number of follicles, small cystic structures each containing an egg, can be seen. The principle is the same as that used by sonar: high-frequency sounds are emitted using a probe inserted into the vagina and, as the nearby organs reflect the sound waves, an image of these organs can be reconstructed. At the beginning of the cycle, five to seven follicles measuring less than 10 millimetres are usually seen in each ovary; in the course of normal ovulation, one of these follicles reaches a size of roughly 20 to 25 millimetres, looking like a "bubble" in the image. The release of the egg can later be confirmed by the disappearance of the dominant follicle, by then completely empty.

Ovarian ultrasound is most often used to 1) indirectly determine the number of good eggs (ovarian reserve assessment) by counting antral follicles; and 2) monitor follicular development triggered by ovulation-inducing agents, especially during assisted reproductive technology procedures (Chapter 5).

CAUSES OF OVULATORY DYSFUNCTION

Identifying ovulatory disorders is important, since several therapeutic approaches are available to correct them. According to the classification proposed by the World Health Organization, there are at least three major groups of ovulatory disorders (a fourth, hyperprolactinemic anovulation, can also be added). Each of these disorders has unique characteristics, stemming both from the underlying causes and from their hormonal profile (figure 23).

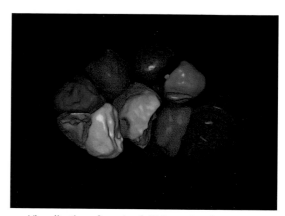

Visualization of ovarian follicles using three-dimensional imaging.

GROUP I: HYPOGONADOTROPIC HYPOGONADAL ANOVULATION

Responsible for approximately 10 percent of anovulation cases, these disorders are most often caused by a breakdown in communication between the hypothalamus and the pituitary, the "command centre" that governs the hormonal cascade involved in ovulation (Chapter 1, pages 24, 26–27). The liberation and pulsatile secretion of gonadotropins (FSH, LH) are severely affected, hindering the normal development and maturation of the ovarian follicles, and are accompanied by a significant decrease in estrogen in the bloodstream, to levels similar to those of menopause. Ovulation does not, therefore, occur, nor does the uterine lining develop, and menstrual periods stop entirely (amenorrhea). In clinical practice, hypoestrogenism caused by this kind of hypothalamic-pituitary insufficiency can be confirmed by administering a drug that mimics the action of progesterone (medroxyprogesterone acetate); the absence of withdrawal bleeding within ten to fourteen days after the progestin is stopped indicates that estrogen levels are too low to support normal endometrial development.

Hypothalamic-pituitary insufficiency is a hormonal imbalance that is sometimes caused by brain pathologies, but can also be the result of a number of extreme behaviours, for example, anorexia or physical over-training.

GROUP II: NORMOGONADOTROPIC NORMOESTROGENIC ANOVULATION

In the vast majority of anovulatory patients (80 percent), the production of pituitary gonadotropins is normal, but their pulsatility, or the frequency with which they are secreted, is not. Blood levels of these hormones, and therefore of estrogen, are high enough to keep the menstrual cycle on track, as evidenced by withdrawal bleeding after administration of a progestin, such as medroxyprogesterone. The problem is therefore less serious than in the case of hypothalamic-pituitary insufficiency (group I). However, despite this apparent normality, ovulation does not occur, or occurs late; patients have menstrual cycles that are too long (> 35 days) or sometimes do not menstruate at all. Various causes can explain these defects in egg maturation.

Hypothalamic Dysfunction

Although not as serious as for anovulation in group I, poor functioning of the hypothalamic-pituitary axis can be responsible for some types of ovulatory dysfunction. These disorders often stem from lifestyle-related factors. For example, unremitting stress, weight loss or gain, or even sustained and very intense physical activity can all negatively affect GnRH secretion and the subsequent release of gonadotropins.

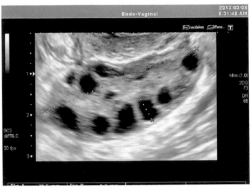

↗ Polycystic ovary (PCOS) visualized by ultrasound.

Polycystic Ovary Syndrome (PCOS)

Described for the first time in 1935, this hormonal disorder must have at least two of the following characteristics:

- Irregular, infrequent, or absent menstrual periods (oligomenorrhea), usually from six to nine periods a year (cycles >35 days).
- High levels of male hormones (biochemical signs of hyperandrogenism) and/or excess facial and body hair (hirsutism), or acne on the face or body (clinical signs of hyperandrogenism).
- Ultrasound confirmation of twelve or more follicles on at least one ovary, measuring from two to nine millimetres in diameter along the ovarian periphery, looking somewhat like a pearl necklace or a rosary. Each cavity is a small immature follicle in which the development and release of the egg are slowed down.

Other rarer causes must be excluded (congenital adrenal hyperplasia, Cushing's disease, an androgen-secreting tumour, etc.).

Despite its widespread prevalence (almost two-thirds of all cases of ovulatory dysfunction), PCOS remains a mysterious disorder, which brings into play a complex mixture of a number of hormonal imbalances. In addition to excess production of androgens by the ovaries, caused by the increased secretion of LH by the pituitary in relation to FSH, PCOS is very often associated with certain metabolic disorders, such as insulin resistance, especially when the patient is overweight or obese. This factor likely plays a key role in the etiology of PCOS, since an elevated insulin level in the ovary interferes with follicle maturation and also stimulates testosterone production, contributing to the side effects typical of too much androgen (hirsutism, acne). This is why certain treatments designed to increase insulin sensitivity (metformin, for example) reset patients' ovulatory cycles and enhance their chances of getting pregnant (see pages 76–77).

GROUP III: HYPERGONADOTROPIC HYPOESTROGENIC ANOVULATION (OVARIAN INSUFFICIENCY)

Also called "premature menopause" or "premature ovarian failure," this serious disorder occurs when the ovaries can no longer synthesize estrogen and produce mature eggs. Ovarian insufficiency is clinically confirmed by a substantial and persistent increase in gonadotropins (FSH and LH), as the pituitary tries to compensate for low estrogen levels by producing an excess of hormones to stimulate estrogen synthesis. These very low levels of estrogen, related to a dramatic decline in the ovarian reserve, cause amenorrhea that persists even when progestin has been administered (absence of withdrawal bleeding). Certain genetic disorders (Fragile X syndrome, gonadal dysgenesis, etc.) and immune disorders, as well as medical (chemotherapy,

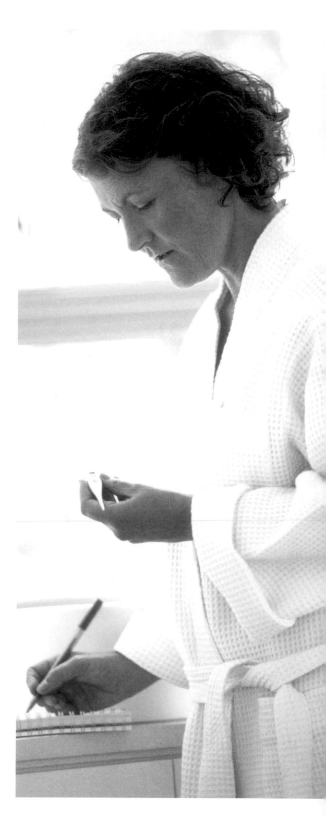

CLASSIFICATION OF OVULATORY DISORDERS ACCORDING TO THE WORLD HEALTH ORGANIZATION

Group	mbnbmnbl	IIa	IIb
	10%	80%	
	Hypogonadotropic hypogonadal anovulation (Hypothalamic-pituitary insufficiency)	Dypothalamic disfunction	Polycystic ovary syndrome
CLINICAL SYMPTOMS	Amenorrhea	Oligomenorrhea or amenorrhea	Oligomenorrhea or amenorrhea Hirsutism, acne
WITHDRAWAL BLEEDING AFTER PROGESTIN	– –	+	+
FSH	N or ↘	N	N
LH	N or ↘	N	N or ↗
ESTRADIOL	↘	N	N or ↗
ANDROGENS (testosterone, DHEAS)	N or ↘	N	N or ↗
OVARIAN RESERVE (antral follicular count)	Variable	N	≥ 12 follicles/ovary (2-9 mm)
MOST COMMON CAUSES	Idiopathic Anorexia Brain tumours and infiltrative lesions Sella turcica syndrome Radiation therapy Kallmann syndrome and other genetic causes Leptin deficiency	Significant weight loss Stress Intense physical exercise Hypothyroidism Obesity Celiac disease	Insulin resistance

N = NORMAL   ↗ = HIGHER   ↘ = LOWER

FIGURE 23

Group	III	Hyperprolactinemic anovulation
	5%	5%
	Ovarian failure Hypergonadotropic hypogonadism (premature menopause)	Hyperprolactinemia
CLINICAL SYMPTOMS	Amenorrhea	Oligomenorrhea or amenorrhea
WITHDRAWAL BLEEDING – AFTER PROGESTIN	–	–/+
FSH	↗	N
LH	↗	N
ESTRADIOL	↘	N or ↘
ANDROGENS (testosterone, DHEAS)	↘	N
OVARIAN RESERVE (antral follicular count)	↘	N
MOST COMMON CAUSES	Genetics (Fragile X syndrome, gonadal dysgenesis) Immune disorders (Savage syndrome) Infections Medical (chemotherapy, radiation therapy)	Prolactin-secreting pituitary adenoma Stress Hypothyroidism Hypothalamic tumour Medications

N = NORMAL   ↗ = HIGHER   ↘ = LOWER

radiotherapy) or surgical procedures are associated with ovarian insufficiency, although, in most cases, the precise reasons for this problem remain unknown. Approximately 6 percent of cases of premature menopause are related to premutations of the FMR1 gene responsible for Fragile X syndrome, and a molecular test is usually conducted when there is a family history of this disorder (early menopause, mental retardation, tremors). Other family members (sisters, for example) may also be screened for this abnormality (FMR1 gene premutations), if the cause is confirmed. A karyotype will usually be prescribed, especially for women under thirty-five, to eliminate other genetic causes. Unfortunately, there is no pharmacological treatment for early menopause, although the use of certain substances such as dehydroepiandrosterone (DHEA) has been suggested. This molecule can cause major side effects, however, and its real effectiveness has not been clearly established. It should only be prescribed under experimental conditions. On the basis of current knowledge, therefore, women who want to have a child have to consider adoption or assisted reproductive technologies using donor eggs. But the issue of fertility aside, women with this disorder must usually take hormone replacement therapy to lessen the risk of osteoporosis as well as heart disease resulting from premature estrogen deficiency.

THYROID DISORDERS

Assessing thyroid gland function can also provide very useful clues as to the causes of anovulation, especially in women who have a family history of thyroid disorders.

In addition to its very significant effects on the metabolism, thyroid influences ovarian function, and a defect in the secretion of hormones by this gland is often associated with an increased risk of infertility and pregnancy loss. Women with this disorder can quickly increase their likelihood of conceiving by taking synthetic thyroid hormones.

HYPERPROLACTINEMIA

Prolactin is the hormone that stimulates milk production by the mammary glands when a newborn sucks on the nipple. In addition to this ancestral physiological mechanism, common to all mammals, the increase in prolactin caused by regularly breastfeeding a child (six to eight times a day) also suppresses ovarian function and thus blocks ovulation most of the time. The effectiveness and duration of this natural contraceptive effect can vary considerably from one woman to another, but it's generally agreed that breastfeeding a child exclusively for the first six months is a way of spacing births.

In addition to breastfeeding, various pathologies can increase blood levels of prolactin and result in anovulation. Certain tumours in the hypothalamic-pituitary region, in particular prolactin adenomas, called prolactinomas, are a frequent cause of hyperprolactinemia. Fortunately, most of these tumours turn out to be benign, and fertility can very often be restored using drugs (bromocriptine, cabergoline) that decrease prolactin secretion and usually get ovulation started again quickly.

TREATMENTS FOR OVULATORY DYSFUNCTION

Treating anovulation calls for restoring the "ovulatory axis," the hormonal cascade linking the brain (hypothalamus and pituitary) to the ovaries, to normal. As of now, there are five main ways to modify this hormonal dynamic (figure 24): 1) anti-estrogens like clomiphene or tamoxifen; 2) aromatase inhibitors like letrozole; 3) improving ovarian response to gonadotropins through metabolic changes (metformin, weight loss); 4) injecting purified or recombinant gonadotropins; and 5) stimulating gonadotropin secretion by administering pulsatile GnRH with a mini-infusion pump.

Which of these treatments are used depends first and foremost on the kinds of hormonal imbalances causing the ovulatory dysfunction (figure 25). However, even when patients' hormonal profiles are similar, the response to these medications may vary greatly from one person to the next, and alternative approaches must often be considered. In every case, the doctor's concern is always to find a delicate balance between stimulating ovulation enough for fertilization to occur and reducing the risk of side effects as much as possible.

ANTIESTROGENS

Given the significant role estrogen plays in the maturing of ovarian follicles, it may at first seem paradoxical to use drugs that neutralize the action of these molecules to trigger ovulation. It must, however, be remembered that the hypothalamic-pituitary-ovarian axis, like all hormonal systems, has an internal regulation mechanism in which the final product (estrogen) controls the departure point of the hormonal cascade (the hypothalamus). While this negative feedback is absolutely essential to prevent the system from getting out of control and producing too much estrogen, it can in some cases hinder the secretion of adequate concentrations of gonadotropins and jeopardize ovulation. By blocking this inhibiting effect, antiestrogens "trick" the brain into believing that estrogen levels are inadequate and that it has to make up for this lack by producing more FSH and LH.

ACTION SITES FOR VARIOUS TREATMENTS FOR OVULATORY DISORDERS

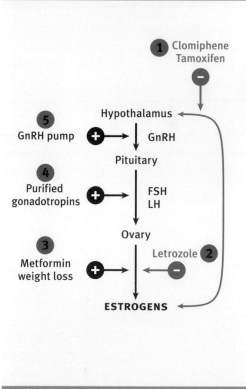

FIGURE 24

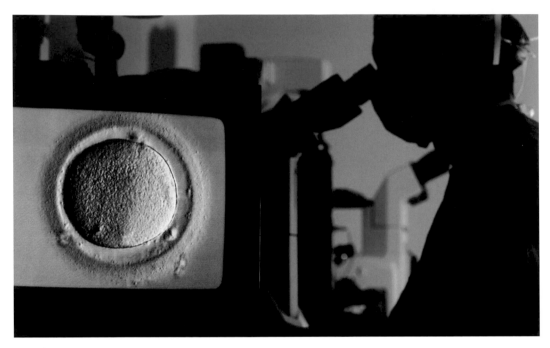

OVERVIEW OF VARIOUS TREATMENTS USED
TO STIMULATE OVARIAN FUNCTION

Causes of anovulation	Patient characteristics	Possible treatments
HYPOTHALAMIC DYSFUNCTION	Normal hormonal profile	Clomiphene Letrozole Tamoxifen
PCOS	Normal weight	Clomiphene Letrozole Tamoxifen
	Excess weight and obesity	Weight loss Metformin Clomiphene/tamoxifen Letrozole
	Clomiphene resistance	Metformin + clomiphene Letrozole ± metformin Gonadotropins
HYPOTHALAMIC PITUITARY INSUFFICIENCY	Clomiphene resistance (negative withdrawal bleeding)	GnRH pump Gonadotropines

FIGURE 25

CHRONIC ANOVULATION (OLIGOMENORRHEA/AMENORRHEA)

Tests : ßhCG, FSH, LH, prolactin, TSH, pelvic ultrasound (ovarian reserve) ± DHEAS, testosterone, AMH, 17-hydroxyprogesterone

Withdrawal bleeding test by administration of medroxyprogesterone acetate (if menstruation has not occurred by day 35 and pregnancy test is negative)

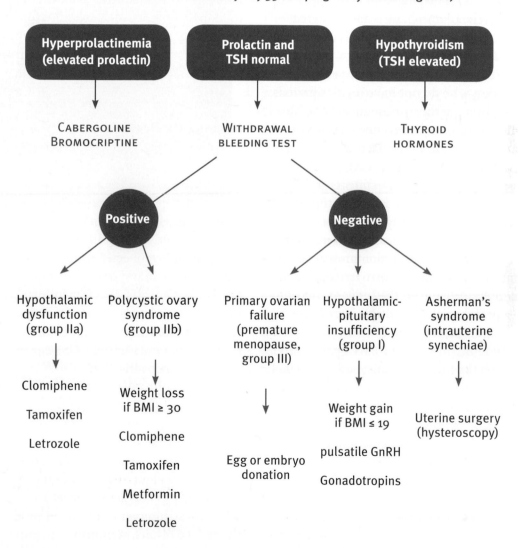

Hyperprolactinemia (elevated prolactin)	Prolactin and TSH normal	Hypothyroidism (TSH elevated)
CABERGOLINE BROMOCRIPTINE	WITHDRAWAL BLEEDING TEST	THYROID HORMONES

Positive

Hypothalamic dysfunction (group IIa)

Clomiphene

Tamoxifen

Letrozole

Polycystic ovary syndrome (group IIb)

Weight loss if BMI ≥ 30

Clomiphene

Tamoxifen

Metformin

Letrozole

Negative

Primary ovarian failure (premature menopause, group III)

Egg or embryo donation

Hypothalamic-pituitary insufficiency (group I)

Weight gain if BMI ≤ 19

pulsatile GnRH

Gonadotropins

Asherman's syndrome (intrauterine synechiae)

Uterine surgery (hysteroscopy)

FIGURE 26

major damage to the tubes, they can accumulate liquid (hydrosalpinx) that interferes with the success of IVF, and the doctor may recommend the tubes be surgically removed before beginning in vitro fertilization procedures.

Tubal blockage is often the result of sexually transmitted infections (STIs) that were not treated in time, mainly chlamydia and gonorrhea. Chlamydia is especially insidious, as this infection is quite widespread, and the bacterium causing it (Chlamydia trachomatis) can do irreversible tubal damage, with few clinical symptoms. The inflammation caused by these infections results in the formation of scar tissue around the pelvic organs that can block the tubal openings. This is why we need to think about our reproductive health even when first becoming sexually active, notably by using condoms during sexual intercourse and, ideally, by limiting the number of partners.

PELVIC FACTORS

Endometriosis

Endometriosis is a disorder in which the cells that make up the uterine lining (endometrium) grow abnormally outside the uterus, most often in the pelvic cavity, on the peritoneum, uterine ligaments, uterine serosa, Fallopian tubes, and ovaries. The unusual outgrowth of endometrial cells and the chronic inflammatory response they cause in the pelvic cavity can result in a wide variety of incapacitating menstrual symptoms (painful periods, abnormal bleeding, ovulatory pain, etc.), as well as various kinds of pain in the pelvic region (painful sexual relations, chronic pelvic pain, etc.). The local release

of inflammatory factors by endometriotic lesions also makes endometriosis harmful to fertility, since extra-uterine endometrial growth may affect both the functioning of the ovaries and Fallopian tubes, and the implantation of the embryo in the uterine lining. The harmful impact of endometriosis is well illustrated by the high prevalence (25 to 50 percent) of this disorder in infertile women, compared with 5 percent in the female population as a whole.

Endometriosis may be treated using laparoscopy, a minimally invasive surgical technique in which a camera and specially adapted surgical instruments (an electrocautery or a laser, for example) are inserted through a small incision in the navel and supra-pubic areas (see the photo of the uterus and its appendages on page 78). Studies show that removing endometrial plaques using this technique leads to a slight but significant increase in the probability of pregnancy, especially if the endometriosis is minimal or mild. Nonetheless, laparoscopy is still an invasive surgical procedure, and its benefits must be carefully weighed against the risks inherent in any operation (general anesthesia, postoperative complications). Unless a patient presents with comorbidities such as endometriotic ovarian cysts (endometriomas) or severe symptoms (painful sexual relations [serious dyspareunia], dysmenorrhea or chronic pelvic pain), it's usually preferable to avoid laparoscopy and try to mitigate the problem by stimulating ovulation with an inducing agent like clomiphene, combined with intrauterine insemination.

Pelvic Adhesions

Adhesions are fibrous tissues that cause the surfaces of normally separate neighbouring tissues to adhere to each other. Several factors can cause pelvic adhesions to form, the most common being inflammatory diseases (peritonitis following the rupture of an abscess on the appendix, Crohn's disease), sexually transmitted diseases, digestive or pelvic operations, and pelvic tuberculosis. The body interprets a lesion on the surface of a tissue to be an injury, which triggers the coagulation system and leads to the formation of a fibrous tissue connecting the damaged tissue to neighbouring structures. The formation of these adhesions is often accompanied by chronic pelvic pain, as well as disruptions in the anatomy of the reproductive system that prevent eggs from moving through the Fallopian tubes and embryos from implanting in the uterus. A number of corrective surgical procedures can be carried out, most often by laparoscopy, but in vitro fertilization often offers a better prognosis.

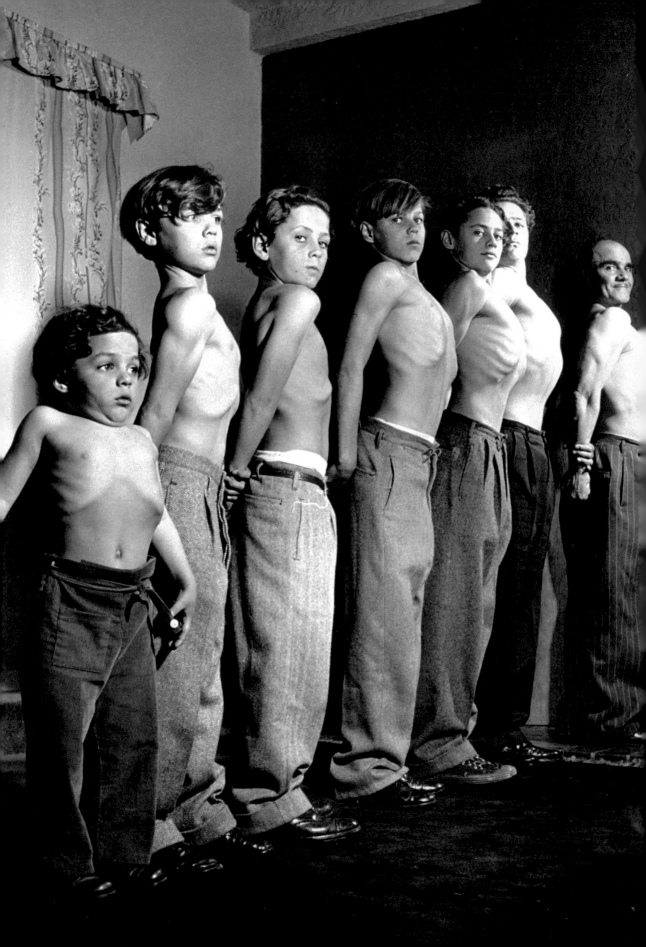

CHAPTER 4

Male Infertility

If you ever feel worthless and depressed, remember:
you were once the fastest sperm of all.
— COLUCHE (1944–1986)

The social perception of masculinity has long been based exclusively on models of physical force, courage, and perseverance. From the first tales boasting of the exploits of ancient heroes (*The Epic of Gilgamesh, The Iliad, The Odyssey*) to the superheroes of our own time, the ideal of a man has very often been that of a being without fear, whose abilities to explore, conquer, and often dominate the world around him compel admiration.

In daily life, this virility was expressed in more practical terms through work, as well as in the functions of "the head of the family." The role of a man, a "real" man, was to work hard to provide for the needs of his wife and family, remaining imperturbable in the face of life's difficulties and being much more comfortable communicating his feelings through his actions than through words. In this kind of context, being able to beget children was an essential aspect of a man's life, allowing him to express his masculinity in a concrete way while playing the role of father assigned to him by society.

While these stereotypes have become more and more out of date and masculinity can now be expressed in very diverse ways, the fact remains that they can still unconsciously influence men's attitudes when infertility is diagnosed. In clinical practice, it's not uncommon for the man's first reaction on being told he is infertile to be disbelief, as he simply can't understand that he could be responsible for the repeated failure of attempts to conceive. Once the first shock has passed, a significant proportion of infertile men can begin to feel that their masculinity is being called into question, and that they are "less masculine" for being unable to perpetuate the family line or fulfil their spouse's desire for a child. Guilt, shame, anger, a feeling of personal failure, and withdrawal into oneself are psychological wounds often observed in infertile men. In the most serious cases, these emotions can result in episodes of depression, anxiety, sleep disturbances, or sexual difficulties.

Yet, while understandable, these reactions do not reflect the reality that infertile men are faced with. Far from being a problem with a person's character or virility, male infertility must first and foremost be considered a medical problem, the result of physiological disorders that upset the production or functioning of sperm and impede their ability to overcome the many barriers separating them from the egg. A diagnosis of infertility, as difficult as it may be to accept, must not be viewed as a sign of weakness, but instead as a well-defined medical condition, and a relatively common one at that, whose causes are becoming better and better understood.

INVESTIGATING MALE INFERTILITY

Since men are in general less likely to consult a doctor about problems related to their reproductive health, many are reluctant and too often postpone participating in the process of investigating fertility. Yet one out of two fertility problems originates in the male, and his participation is absolutely indispensable for deciding which medical procedures are most likely to improve the chances of successful conception.

Physical Assessment

A complete fertility work-up usually includes a physical examination of the patient. Obviously, particular attention is paid to the genital organs: the testicles are palpated to measure their volume, as well as the continuity of the genitourinary tract (head, body, and tail of the epididymis, vas deferens), while in some cases prostatitis can be detected by means of a digital rectal examination. Secondary sexual characteristics like overall stature, hairiness, and mammary development (gynecomastia) are also evaluated. These observations, combined with a comprehensive interview to review the patient's medical history (infections, metabolic diseases, lifestyle habits, etc.) enable the doctor to identify a number of diagnostic leads that can later be confirmed using more precise tests.

SEMEN ANALYSIS

Fertility problems originating in the male can usually be diagnosed quickly by a semen analysis, which studies the main sperm parameters (sperm count, motility, and shape), as well as those of the semen (volume, pH, white blood cell count) (figure 28). This is very often the first test prescribed for couples who visit a doctor because they have not been able to conceive, since, compared with the procedures used to investigate female infertility, the production of a semen sample does not require an invasive or painful examination and can be done several times over in a short span of time.

The procedure essentially involves observing a sample of semen through a microscope with a camera that is able to capture images and send them to a computer for analysis. In a way, this is the modern version of the slide used by Dutchman Antonie van Leeuwenhoek over three hundred years ago (see page 88).

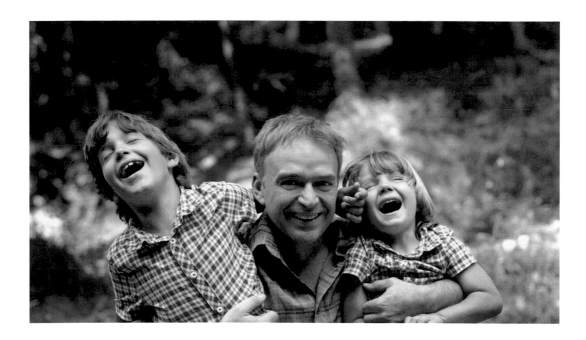

THE VARIOUS SEMEN PARAMETERS
EVALUATED BY MEANS OF A SPERMOGRAM

Parameter	Lower reference limit
Volume of semen (ml)	1.5
Total number of sperm cells (10^6 in the ejaculate)	39
Concentration of sperm (10^6 per ml)	15
Total motility (PR + NP, %)	40
Progressive motility (PR, %)	32
Vitality (live sperm, %)	58
Sperm morphology (normal shapes, %)	4
Other threshold values accepted	
pH	≥ 7.2
Peroxidase-positive leucocytes (10^6 per ml)	< 1.0
Antibody antisperm test (%)	< 50

PR = PROGRESSIVE   NP = NON-PROGRESSIVE

FIGURE 28   Source: Adapted from NHS Foundation Trust (United Kingdom), 2013 and Cooper et al., 2010.

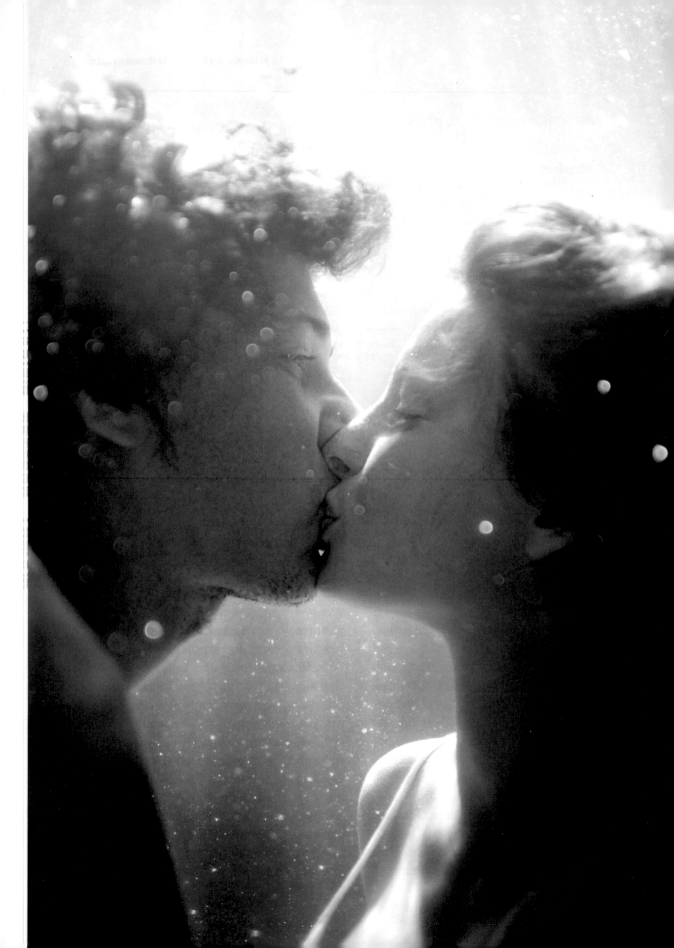

CHAPTER 5

Assisted Reproductive Technologies

Now we two, smiling at the evening star,
Felt the bright gleams of hope rise up once more [...][4]
— ÉMILE NELLIGAN (1879–1941)

For many couples, starting a family is one of life's most important priorities, the culmination of a dream that is a key part of a full and successful life. Faced with the hard reality of seeing this desire unfulfilled, individuals who are infertile can lose their bearings, completely call into question their sincerest values, and come to view their lives as a major failure. There is hope, however: the remarkable progress made in recent decades by modern medicine means that more and more infertile people manage to overcome this disease and achieve their desire to have a child. In addition to actually saving lives, human ingenuity can also play a major role in the very conception of life, by intervening actively to help make sure the cellular events necessary for fertilization take place.

INTRAUTERINE INSEMINATION

Homologous intrauterine insemination (IUI) (with the partner's sperm) is a simple and painless assisted reproductive procedure that can be used in five main situations.

- Infertility whose cause remains unexplained, despite thorough investigation (semen analysis, ovulatory profile, and tubal permeability all normal).
- Infertility related to minimal or mild endometriosis, with at least one permeable tube.
- Mild or moderate male infertility, with reduced concentration or motility of sperm, but with at least a million sperm per millilitre.
- Infertility resulting from the absence of sexual relations, owing to physical problems (for example, erectile dysfunction, paraplegia) or certain psychogenic causes.

• Infertility caused by a cervical factor (for example, previous surgery on the cervix).

The principle of IUI is relatively simple: it's a matter of depositing a sufficient quantity of motile sperm directly inside the uterus, in the hope they will then travel through the tubes and fertilize an egg (figure 35). While less technically demanding than other assisted reproductive procedures, insemination requires a rigorous approach to control the two parameters essential for its success.

The Timing of Insemination

It goes without saying that insemination must be carried out as close to ovulation as possible to maximize the chances of fertilization. There are two ways to determine this with greatest accuracy.

The simplest is to take an ovulation test: available in drugstores and superstores, these tests detect the increase in LH levels in the urine that occurs from 24 to 36 hours before ovulation and can often make it possible to estimate the time when the egg can be fertilized. To make sure the increase in LH in the urine is not missed,

INTRAUTERINE INSEMINATION

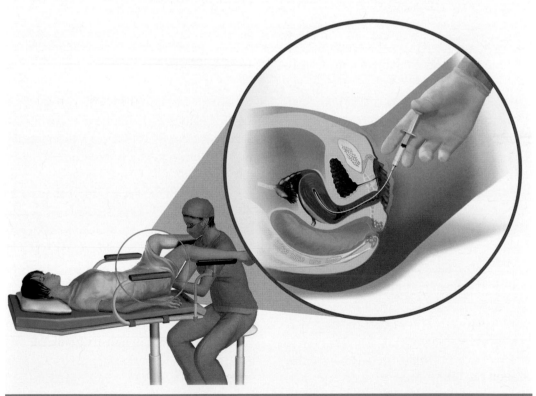

FIGURE 35

the procedures must be started approximately four days before the anticipated day of ovulation; for example, for a 28-day menstrual cycle, the critical pre-ovulatory period begins around day 10 of the cycle (the 10th day after the beginning of the period). The test is conducted on the second urine sample of the day, ideally between 7:00 and 7:30 a.m., by dipping the stick into urine collected in a container (it's also possible, with some tests, to urinate directly onto the stick). Depending on the manufacturer, a colour, line, or "plus" sign appears, indicating that the amount of LH is increasing and that ovulation should occur in the following 24 to 36 hours. The patient must then immediately contact the clinic to make an appointment for insemination.

The other option is to take a series of ultrasounds, repeated at regular intervals during the pre-ovulatory period, so as to watch the ovarian follicles mature. When a dominant follicle reaches around 18 to 25 millimetres in size, chorionic gonadotropin hormone (CGH) is prescribed to artificially trigger ovulation, and an appointment is made for the next day to carry out the insemination. This ultrasound monitoring is especially important when the ovarian response is induced or stimulated using "superovulants," such as gonadotropins, as it makes it possible to see the number of follicles that are developing during the treatment. If the ultrasound indicates that there are from one to three dominant follicles, CGH is administered to induce ovulation, instead of endogenous LH, and insemination can take place. On the other hand, if more than three or four follicles have developed, the risk of multiple pregnancy becomes considerably higher and either the insemination procedure is cancelled, or it

is turned into an in vitro fertilization procedure, in which the number of embryos transferred can be controlled (see page 100).

Preparing the Sperm
The major advantage of IUI is that sperm can get through the cervix without hindrance, thus taking a "giant step" in their journey to the egg. To manage this, however, there must be a sufficient quantity of sperm and they must be in "good shape," with enough motility to enable them to travel through the tubes in hopes of fertilizing an egg at the end. Proper preparation of the sperm is therefore of prime importance for the insemination to succeed.

A semen sample must be produced by the male partner on the same day as the insemination, preferably at the clinic where the procedure will be carried out. The specimen can also be produced at home, but in that case very careful attention must be paid (especially in winter) to maintaining it at body temperature, by placing it in the armpit, for example. As soon as the sample is received, the semen is centrifuged to eliminate impurities (dead cells, white blood cells) as well as the seminal fluid surrounding the sperm. Without this preparation, the direct injection of semen would trigger intense uterine contractions due to the prostaglandins it contains, expose the woman to a greater risk of pelvic infection, and potentially harm the sperm's chances of getting into the tubes. Using density gradient preparation, the best sperm are selected and can then be used for insemination. Generally speaking, at least 500,000 to 1,000,000 motile sperm must be injected into the uterine cavity to increase the probability of achieving a pregnancy.

Intrauterine insemination has higher chances of success when combined with ovulatory stimulation. This raises the monthly pregnancy rate with IUI to approximately 10 to 13 percent, comparing favourably with couples' chances of conceiving naturally (2 to 3 percent per month). Roughly half of women under forty get pregnant during the first six cycles of intrauterine insemination, a result significantly higher than that obtained using ovulation agents alone. When intrauterine insemination does not succeed in yielding positive results after three to six cycles, in vitro fertilization must then be considered. In a more aggressive and efficient approach, the National Institute for Health and Care Excellence (UK) recently advised that for people with unexplained infertility, mild endometriosis or mild male infertility trying to conceive for a total of at least two years, IVF should, from now on, be offered as a first line therapy, bypassing IUI.

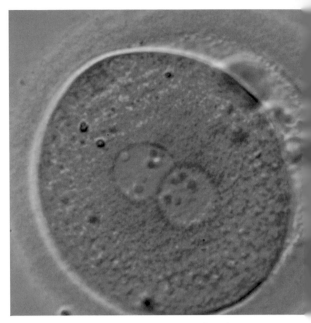

↗ In vitro fertilization using intracytoplasmic sperm injection.

IN VITRO FERTILIZATION

After having been the subject of heated debate in its early years, in vitro fertilization is now considered to be one of the greatest success stories of modern medicine, a success recognized by the awarding of the Nobel Prize in medicine to Robert Edwards in 2010. Far from being a danger to children's health or a springboard to the mass production of "artificial children," as some feared at the beginning, these procedures have on the contrary become accepted over the years as an effective treatment for many infertile couples, with more than five million children having been born since the birth of Louise Brown in July 1978.

In the popular imagination, children born following in vitro fertilization have long been nicknamed "test-tube babies," an image that may imply that their birth was due to a completely artificial process that took place entirely outside their mother's body. Obviously, this is not the case! In reality, the goal of in vitro fertilization is not to be a substitute for the natural process of conception, but simply to facilitate it, to overcome certain physiological disorders that prevent sperm from making contact with the egg. The strategy is mainly used to treat the following conditions:

- Total blockage of the tubes, which can't be corrected by surgery or has a poor surgical prognosis.
- Severe male infertility, i.e. semen with fewer than a million sperm per

millilitre; total absence of sperm in the semen, even though there are sperm in the testicles (ejaculatory duct blockage, defective spermatogenesis following infection, cancer treatment, an idiopathic cause, etc.). An epididymal or testicular sampling is then required.

- Moderate or severe endometriosis, mechanically making it more difficult to conceive with simpler treatments.
- Failure to conceive after a total of two years, in people with unexplained infertility, mild endometriosis, or mild male infertility.
- Failure to conceive despite treatments such as ovulation-inducing agents, endometriosis or tubal treatments, and intrauterine insemination.
- A loss of ovarian function owing to cancer treatment, using cryopreserved eggs.

The general principle of in vitro fertilization is relatively simple: it involves removing eggs produced by the patient after having stimulated ovarian function with drugs, fertilizing them in the laboratory with sperm to create embryos, and then introducing a certain number of these embryos (ideally just one) into the uterus, in the hope that it will implant successfully.

In fact, in vitro fertilization is a complex procedure, calling on a number of medical procedures that can make the experience emotionally and physically demanding. However, it is possible to approach this challenge confidently and calmly by taking a broad view of the medical approach being taken, as well as by better understanding the objective and the importance of the medical procedures that will be followed throughout the process. What's more,

new innovations such as removing an egg during natural cycles could someday simplify in vitro fertilization even more and as a result make it less intimidating.

FIVE STEPS TO MAKING A BABY

STEP 1: STIMULATING OVULATION

Despite the considerable technical advances made in recent decades, IVF remains a procedure with an average success rate of just 30 percent per attempt (per menstrual cycle). This success rate is comparable to monthly fertility rates in fertile couples, but the high proportion of failures remains problematic, given the cost of the procedure and the physical demands on the patient. To make up for these limitations, a commonly used strategy is to trigger the simultaneous maturation of several eggs during the same cycle, the idea being to obtain enough embryos to be able to select and implant the one or ones most likely to result in a successful pregnancy. However, this "superovulation" can cause various side effects (see box page 103) and much effort has been devoted in recent years to simplifying the stimulation protocol, by developing "gentler" versions in which IVF is carried out using very mild ovarian stimulation or without medication during the patient's natural cycle. Three simplified methods have been proposed: 1) IVF with mild ovarian stimulation; 2) IVF done during an entirely natural cycle, without ovarian stimulation; 3) modified natural IVF (figure 36). These three approaches have several advantages over classic IVF, among them a substantially lower cost for drugs and the total or near total absence of the

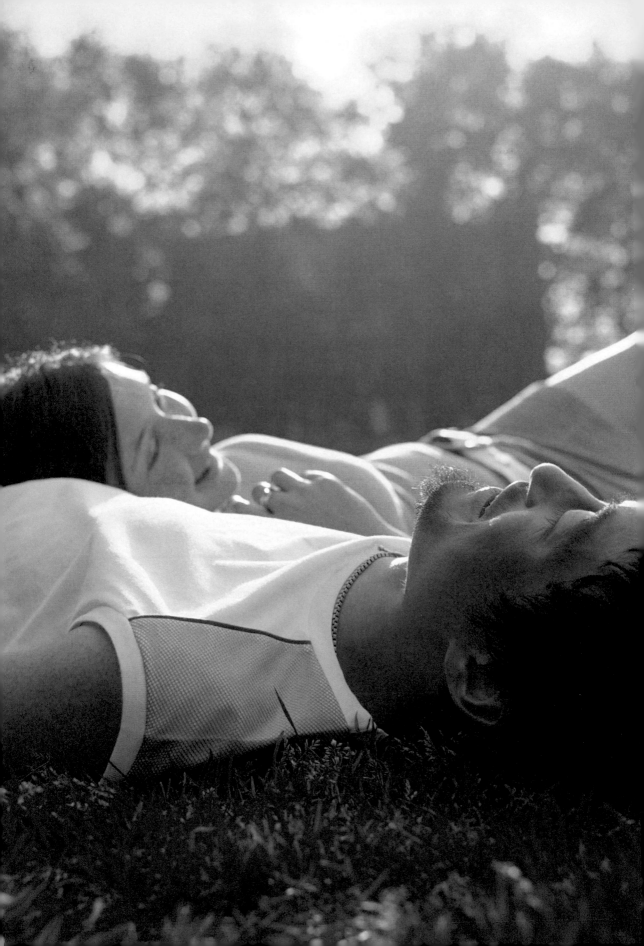

syndromes of ovarian hyperstimulation and multiple pregnancies. However, each of these approaches has its own advantages and disadvantages, and the choice of one or the other of these procedures is usually made based on the cause of the infertility, the couple's age, and their own preference.

Classic IVF

In most clinical protocols, "superovulation" is achieved by administering high doses of the gonadotropin FSH or hMG (a combination of FSH and LH). These hormones promote the development of all follicles that have reached a sufficiently advanced stage of maturation, usually allowing between eight and twelve eggs to be retrieved, depending on the dose prescribed. Because of the powerful action of these gonadotropins, superovulation requires close medical monitoring, during which the growth of the follicles is observed using ultrasounds repeated at regular intervals.

The simultaneous maturation of several follicles causes the amount of estrogen to increase considerably, which normally results in the secretion of LH to induce ovulation. To prevent this situation from occurring, superovulation treatments are preceded by the administration of drugs (GnRH agonists) that exhaust the supply

VARIOUS PROTOCOLS THAT CAN BE USED TO INDUCE OVULATION IN AN IN VITRO FERTILIZATION PROCEDURE

Type of IVF	Goal	Drugs and hormones used
Classic IVF (conventional)	≥ 8 eggs	GnRH agonist (leuprolide, buserelin, nafarelin, triptorelin) GnRH antagonist (Cetrotide, ganirelix)
Mild IVF	2 to 7 eggs	Gonadotropins (FSH/hMG: follicle Oral agents (clomiphene, letrozole) GnRH antagonist (low dose) Gonadotropins (low dose)
IVF in a modified natural cycle	1 egg	GnRH antagonist (low dose) GnRH antagonist (low dose)
IVF in a natural cycle	1 egg	None

FIGURE 36

of gonadotropins in the pituitary gland and prevent it from producing more. The pronounced decrease in endogenous FSH and LH puts the ovaries into a stationary condition before the stimulation stage, while preventing any spontaneous release of eggs when follicle growth is induced using gonadotropins.

In what is called the "long IVF protocol," ovarian function is suppressed by administering GnRH agonists, starting two to three weeks before beginning ovarian stimulation using gonadotropins (day 21 of the preceding cycle or at the onset of the period) (figure 37). This approach resets ovarian function and usually results in a good response to the subsequent gonadotropin treatment. However, the significant decrease in estrogen production that occurs during the temporary pause in ovarian function causes symptoms typical of menopause (hot flashes, headaches, vaginal

SEQUENCE OF TREATMENTS USED IN VARIOUS IV FERTILIZATION PROTOCOLS

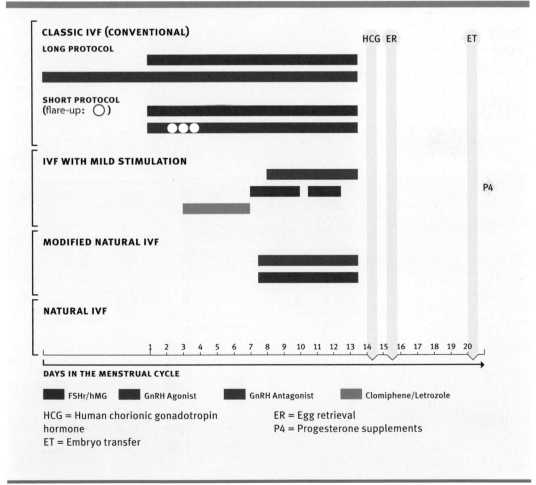

FIGURE 37

dryness) and this can be uncomfortable for the patient. In some so-called "short protocols," GnRH agonists are given at the beginning of the cycle, right before gonadotropins. This prevents spontaneous ovulation, while reducing the side effects associated with suppressing the ovaries. This short protocol is mainly used in women who do not respond as well to gonadotropins.

All of these hormonal manipulations make ovarian stimulation one of the longest and most uncomfortable stages in the classic IVF cycle, both because of the number of drugs used and their undesirable side effects. One of reproductive medicine's major concerns is, therefore, to simplify ovarian stimulation procedures as much as possible to make them less harsh and restrictive for patients.

IVF with Mild Ovarian Stimulation

Mild (or minimal) ovarian stimulation is increasingly preferred by some medical teams, both for women with a low egg reserve and for those who are at risk of responding too strongly to gonadotropins (polycystic ovary syndrome, in particular). It may also be considered as a first-line treatment for all couples. This procedure consists of stimulating the ovaries using anti-estrogens like clomiphene or letrozole (see page 104), followed or not by the administration of low doses of gonadotropins. To prevent premature ovulation, a GnRH antagonist is usually added when the dominant follicle reaches 14 millimetres in diameter and administered until the eggs are retrieved, usually from two to seven days later.

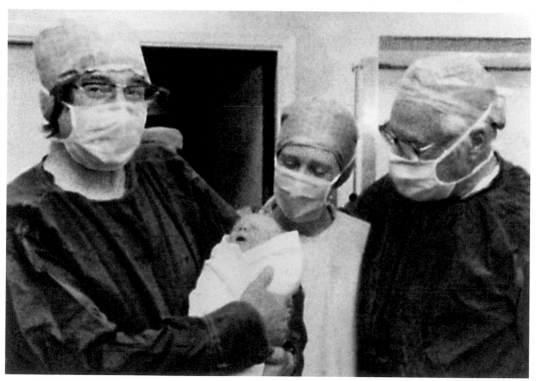

↗ First birth resulting from IVF, in 1978, that of Louise Brown. From left to right, Robert Edwards, Jean Purdy, and Patrick Steptoe.

IVF in a Natural Cycle

The first IVF birth (Louise Brown, in 1978) resulted from a natural cycle, unstimulated in other words, during which a single egg is usually produced. However, owing to its many initial failures, "natural" IVF was considered to be very ineffective and was soon abandoned in favour of IVF using stimulated cycles. The protocol for IVF in a natural cycle is quite simple, since it neither requires the administration of gonadotropins nor GnRH agonists, and blood tests to measure estradiol are seldom necessary. Ultrasound monitoring begins only around the seventh day of the cycle so as to monitor the growth of the dominant follicle and the development of the uterine lining. A dominant ovarian follicle 16 millimetres or more in diameter is used as the criterion to trigger ovulation.

IVF in a Modified Natural Cycle

A modified natural cycle aims to prevent LH, the hormone that gets the ovulation process underway, from peaking prematurely, and to support the final development of the dominant follicle for several days. Once it has been determined that there are no ovarian cysts, the ultrasound monitoring of follicular growth starts on the sixth day of the cycle (for a 28-day cycle) and, as soon as the dominant follicle reaches 14 millimetres in diameter, a GnRH antagonist is administered to prevent spontaneous ovulation. The administration of gonadotropins also begins, at the same time every day.

For certain categories of patient with a favourable prognosis, the pregnancy rate of 23 percent per modified natural cycle appears to be comparable to that achieved using IVF with classic ovarian stimulation (24 percent), but which requires GnRH agonists and on average more than twenty times as much gonadotropin.

Step 2: Retrieving the Eggs

Regardless of the ovarian stimulation protocol used, when the ultrasound shows follicles that are big enough (from 18 to 25 millimetres), the final maturation of the eggs is completed using a single injection of hCG. Acting not unlike LH, this hormone enables the egg to gradually detach itself from the follicle wall and, if egg retrieval does not take place, to be released into the pelvic cavity 36 to 39 hours later; so as not to "lose" eggs, the retrieval must therefore be done approximately 35 to 36 hours after the hCG injection, before spontaneous ovulation occurs. In practice, this means that hCG is usually injected in the evening, so that retrieval can be carried out two days later, just before the eggs are released. Eggs are retrieved through the vagina, using a fine needle connected to an ultrasound probe that helps visualize the follicles. This is a delicate procedure, usually carried out under sedation (sometimes under local anesthetic), which involves perforating the follicles with the needle and aspirating the liquid they contain to recover the eggs within.

The number of eggs retrieved will obviously depend on the stimulation protocol used: in classic IVF, superovulation allows several follicles to develop and ten eggs on average to be retrieved. This number is lower in IVF with mild stimulation (between two and seven), but is still high enough to achieve pregnancy rates approaching those of classic IVF (between 23 and 43 percent per attempt), even in women who've had repeated IVF failures.

From left to right, from top to bottom: non-fertilized egg; four-cell embryo (approximately 40 to 48 hours after fertilization); eight-cell embryos (approximately 72 hours after fertilization); morula (16 to 32 cells); blastocysts (⸺⸽ 64 cells). ↗

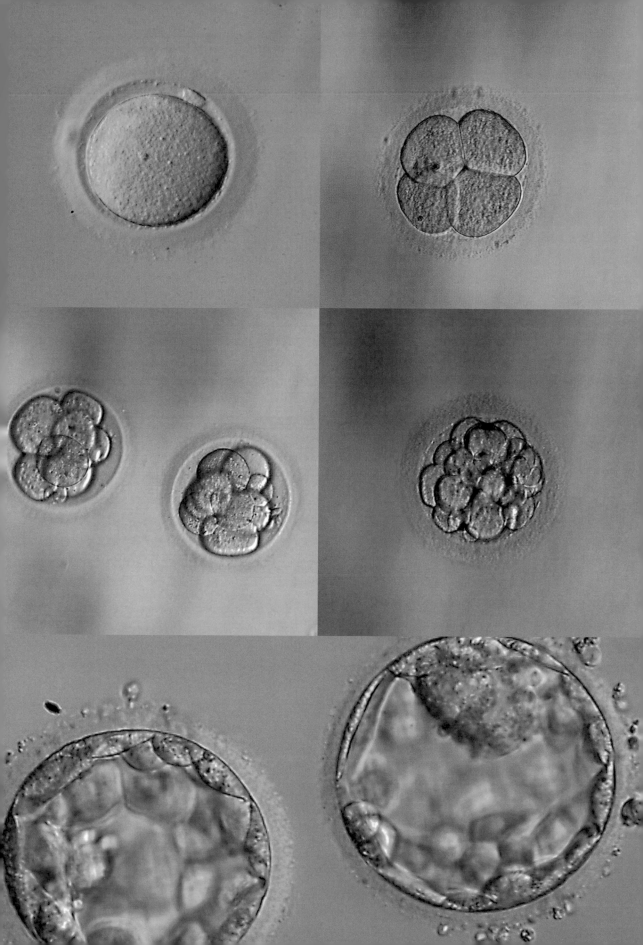

With these protocols, the vast majority of patients will have at least one embryo transferred.

As for IVF in natural cycles, a high rate of failure (20 to 25 percent) in retrieving the egg is the most common problem. Various causes may explain this, including follicular atresia or premature ovulation before retrieval. Only 50 to 60 percent of women will have, in a natural cycle, an embryo transfer per attempt; a success rate of 7 to 10 percent per start of treatment and 16 to 18 percent per embryo transfer can be hoped for. The effectiveness of this treatment is therefore debatable. The pregnancy rates may, however, prove to be higher in certain couples, especially younger ones.

STEP 3: FERTILIZATION

Fertilization in a Conventional Laboratory The same day the eggs are retrieved, a sperm preparation is made using a sample of semen produced by the partner. A period of abstinence of two to five days ahead of time is usually recommended, to encourage sperm to accumulate and thus produce the best possible sample. The next step in the process is relatively simple: it's just a matter of placing each of the eggs harvested in a small plastic dish (a Petri dish), adding 50,000 to 100,000 motile sperm, and letting fertilization take its course by keeping the boxes for several hours in a temperature and atmosphere equivalent to that of the human body. Around 16 to 18 hours after the addition of the sperm, the fertilization of the egg can easily be seen under the microscope in the form of two adjacent circles, containing the genetic material from the egg and sperm that are about to fuse.

ICSI

In cases of severe male infertility, the laboratory fertilization stage is more complex. When the sperm are few in number, lacking, or have too little motility, one sperm cell must be isolated and injected right into the egg, using a small glass needle guided by a microscope.

This sperm micro-injection technique (intracytoplasmic sperm injection, or ICSI), first used successfully in 1992, is a major technological breakthrough for male infertility. It can be done using the few sperm present in the semen, or even when there are none in the ejaculate (azoospermia). When this is the case, a prior step is to surgically retrieve mature sperm from the epididymis (obstructive azoospermia, caused by a defect in excretion) or immature sperm from the testicles (non-obstructive azoospermia, caused by a defect in maturation). While delicate, ICSI is a procedure with an excellent fecundity rate (75 percent of eggs are fertilized) and it now means that many couples can have a biological child instead of having to turn to insemination with donor sperm or adoption.

Technological advances continue. For example, in order to improve even more the success rates of ICSI, some have recently suggested choosing sperm based on their morphology using high-magnification microscopy (IMSI).

STEP 4: IMPLANTING THE EMBRYOS

As with fertilization, the first stages of embryonic development can be re-created in vitro, by placing the fertilized eggs in an environment containing all the ingredients required for cell division. The embryo begins to develop around 24 hours after the fusion of the genetic material in the egg and sperm, becoming approximately 4 cells after 2 days and 8 cells after 3 days, at which point their development has advanced enough for them to be transferred into the uterus. Embryo transfer consists of inserting a thin and flexible plastic tube into the vagina and depositing the embryo or embryos that have been developing for between 2 and 5 days in the laboratory into the uterine cavity, using an ultrasound guide when necessary. This procedure only lasts a few minutes and is usually painless. Furthermore, contrary to what we might think, patients are not told to limit their activities in the days after the transfer; studies show that rest might even be harmful.

Depending on the number of eggs fertilized in the laboratory, they can sometimes be allowed to develop until the fifth day so they can reach the blastocyst stage (approximately one hundred cells). Only the strongest embryos reach this stage; implanting blastocysts increases the implantation rate per embryo considerably, and thus the chances of getting pregnant.

The most important parameter in the implantation stage remains, however, the number of embryos transferred. In classic IVF, where fertilizing from eight to twelve eggs makes it possible to obtain several high- quality embryos, it used to be common to implant two or three separate embryos (and sometimes more) to increase the likelihood of pregnancy; this approach had the major disadvantage of dramatically increasing the number of at-risk multiple pregnancies. Over the years, a growing determination to reduce the incidence of multiple pregnancies has led to a re-evaluation of implantation protocols. In

Quebec, for example, the IVF program stipulates the transfer of a single embryo in the majority of cases, with the result being a noticeable drop in multiple pregnancies.

In addition to significantly reducing the risk of multiple pregnancy, single embryo transfer has a positive impact on the likelihood of the child being born in good health (figure 38). At all maternal ages, implanting a single embryo cuts in half the proportion of children born with a handicap and, even more important, perinatal mortality (death after 28 weeks' gestation or shortly after birth). This is an extremely important statistic, for the ultimate objective of IVF is not to conceive children at any cost, but rather to make sure that these children are born in good health and live the longest and healthiest lives possible.

A significant decrease is seen in the incidence of twins and perinatal mortality following single transfer, at all maternal ages.

The emphasis on transferring a single embryo is all the more important since the success rates for IVF are comparable to those obtained when two embryos are transferred, in the neighbourhood of 30 to 40 percent of live births after six cycles (figure 40). In case of failure, the extra embryos of high quality that were not implanted can be frozen and transferred later, during natural cycles, without repeating the initial steps in the procedure (ovarian stimulation and egg retrieval). For women over forty, on the other hand, transferring a single embryo does not usually result in a satisfactory pregnancy rate and two embryos are still implanted, despite the high increase in risk (twenty times) of twins.

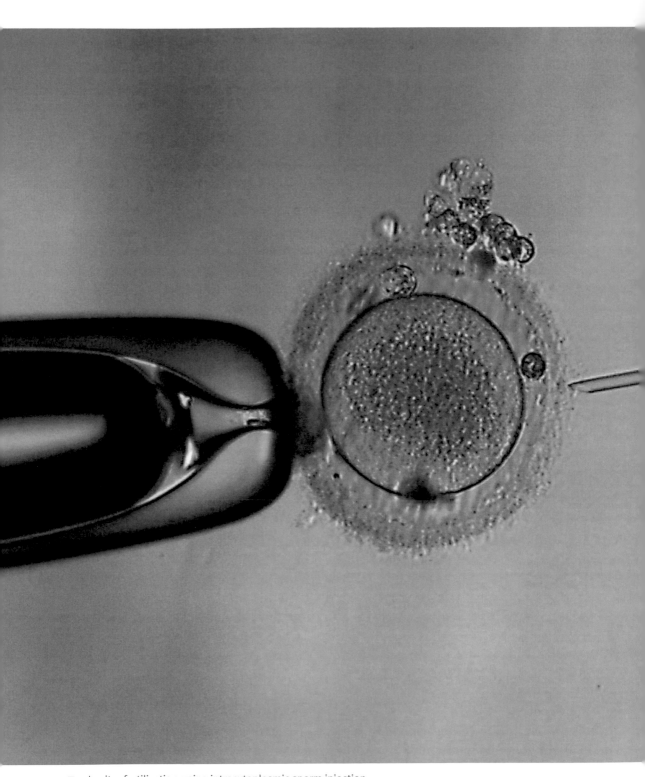

↗   In vitro fertilization using intracytoplasmic sperm injection.

STEP 5: THE LUTEAL PHASE AND PREGNANCY

During the luteal phase of a normal menstrual cycle, progesterone secretion by the corpus luteum gradually makes the uterine lining more receptive to the fertilized embryo (Chapter 1, page 31). Supraphysiological blood hormone levels produced by ovarian stimulation in classic IVF would cause disruptions in the luteal phase and lessen the endometrium's receptivity to the embryo. Progesterone supplements must therefore be administered as soon as the embryos are transferred, to encourage their implantation. The progesterone is usually administered vaginally as tablets, suppositories, or gels, or sometimes parenterally (intramuscularly). However, no study indicates that it's useful to continue administering progesterone past the sixth week of pregnancy, once the viability of the pregnancy is confirmed by ultrasound.

Despite its complexity and limitations, in vitro fertilization is nonetheless an effective assisted reproductive technology procedure, with a success rate comparable to that of fertile couples. And even when the first try proves unsuccessful, the likelihood of conceiving during subsequent attempts remains very high, so much so that a significant proportion of women can expect to get pregnant after three to six cycles of IVF. Furthermore, the constant improvement in techniques, notably the development of milder ovarian stimulation protocols, has resulted in many fewer side effects, as well as lower drug costs. This really is a medical revolution, enabling infertile couples to finally fulfil their desire to start a family.

RATES OF LIVE BIRTHS OBTAINED USING CLASSIC IVF (BLUE) OR IVF WITH MILD STIMULATION (RED)

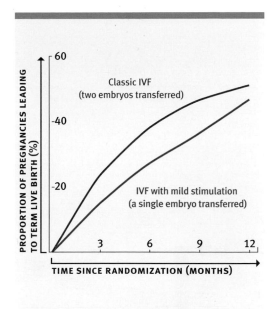

FIGURE 38

IMPACT OF ELECTIVE SINGLE EMBRYO TRANSFER PER IVF CYCLE DIRECTIVE (QUEBEC PROGRAM)

	Before	After
eSET (%)	1.6%	49%
Clinical pregnancies (%/ET)	42.7%	31%
Multiple pregnancies (%)	27.2%	5.2%

ET = Embryo transfer
eSET = elective single-embryo transfer or SET (single embryo transfer)

FIGURE 39

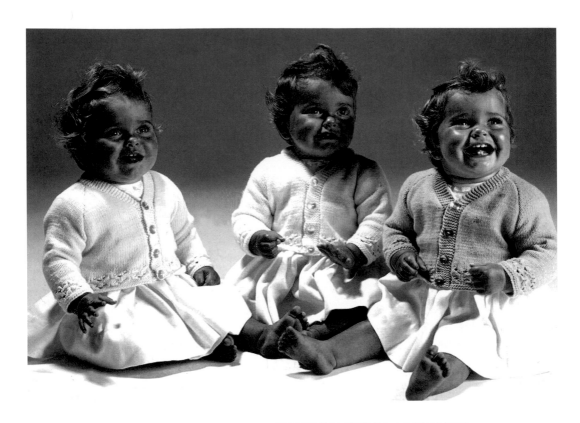

CUMULATIVE LIVE BIRTH RATE AFTER THREE IVF CYCLES ACCORDING TO THE NUMBER OF EMBRYOS TRANSFERRED PER CYCLE

Woman's age	32 years		36 years		39 years	
Transfer strategy	eSET	DET	eSET	DET	eSET	DET
Live births (%)	50.4	58.5*	40.5	47.4*	29.4	37.1*
Full-term births (%)	45.4	46.8	36.4	38.6	26.5	30.9*
Single child births (%)	48.9*	40.2	39.3*	34.3	28.7	28.7
Twin births (%)	2.5	27.6*	2.3	23.4*	1.9	19.1*
Handicap (out of 1,000 births)	7.5	14.0*	6.0	10.5*	4.3	7.7*
Perinatal deaths (out of 1,000 births)	5.0	10.6*	4.0	8.0*	2.9	5.8*

* Significant to p = 0.05

eSET = elective single-embryo transfer
DET = double-embryo transfer

FIGURE 40

Source: Adapted from Scotland et al., 2011.

QUESTIONS FREQUENTLY ASKED BY PATIENTS STARTING A MEDICALLY ASSISTED REPRODUCTIVE PROCEDURE

Is a Diagnostic Laparoscopy Required Before IVF?

Laparoscopy may be indicated if there are pelvic disorders, such as dilated Fallopian tubes (hydrosalpinx), ovarian cysts, or severe endometriosis symptoms. A previous IVF failure may also point to the usefulness of a laparoscopic examination. On the other hand, laparoscopy is usually avoided when a cause of infertility has been identified (especially male infertility), there are no suspected clinical symptoms, and a pelvic ultrasound is normal.

Do Uterine Fibroids Have to Be Removed Before IVF?

Uterine fibroids on the external uterine wall (sub-serous) do not seem to have a negative effect on fertility and they should only be removed if they are symptomatic. As for fibroids in the muscle (intramural), while they are associated with decreased fertility and an increase in miscarriages, available scientific data do not confirm the usefulness of a resection (myomectomy) for improving the success rates of assisted reproductive technologies. In the case of fibroids protruding into the uterine cavity, there appears to be a clinical advantage in removing them before IVF, usually using hysteroscopy, in order to improve the success rate.

Do Endometrial Polyps Have to Be Removed Before IVF?

Scientific studies are divided over the effect

Ovarian Hyperstimulation Syndrome

Ovarian hyperstimulation syndrome is rare (it occurs in approximately 1 percent of cases), but it can nonetheless have serious repercussions for the patient's health. This complication from superovulation takes the form of multiple follicular cysts, formed by an abnormal accumulation of liquid, that develop following egg retrieval. The first symptoms are usually substantial and rapid abdominal bloating, often accompanied by cramps in the lower part of the abdomen, nausea and weight gain. Ovarian hyperstimulation is usually mild; the abdominal discomfort does not last long, but can in some cases reach a dangerous clinical stage: when there is a significant accumulation of liquid in the abdomen (ascites) and the lungs (hydrothorax), blood hyperviscosity, and acute renal failure, the patient's condition may deteriorate rapidly, putting her life in danger. For all of these reasons, gonadotropins are always administered under the close supervision of a doctor, and the procedure is immediately stopped if there are any clinical signs that might suggest an increased risk of ovarian hyperstimulation.

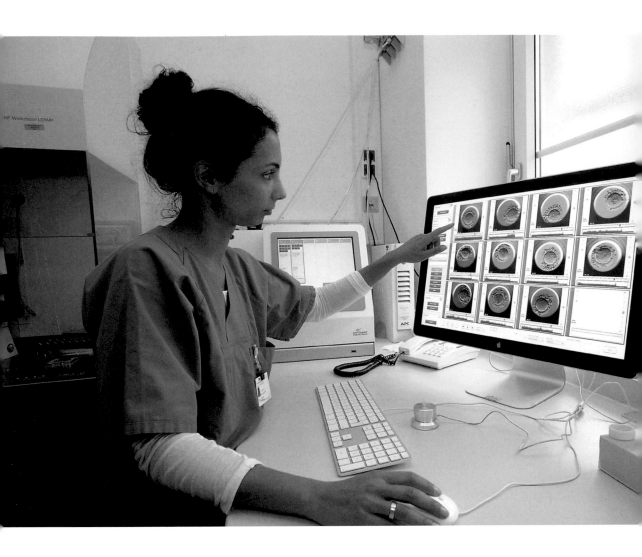

of polyps and their extraction on fertility. Endometrial polypectomy is, however, a fairly minor low-risk surgical procedure; removing endometrial polyps before IVF is, therefore, recommended.

Do Vitamin Supplements Improve IVF Success Rates?

Folic acid supplementation before and during pregnancy significantly reduces the risk of open neural tube defects in the fetus. As for other vitamin supplements, no sufficiently complete data are available to warrant recommending that they be prescribed as part of IVF, for either women or men. A healthy diet is always recommended.

Is There Any Reason to Administer Metformin Before IVF in Patients with Polycystic Ovary Syndrome?

Current scientific evidence supports the use of metformin in patients with polycystic ovaries. Although the drug does not necessarily increase the birth rate following IVF, it significantly lowers the risk of ovarian hyperstimulation syndrome.

Who Could Benefit from Invitro Egg Maturation?

In vitro egg maturation is a relatively recent technology, in which immature eggs are retrieved and brought to maturity in a laboratory. It does not require the use of ovulation-inducing agents and can be offered to patients at high risk of developing ovarian hyperstimulation syndrome.

Women whose response to ovarian stimulation is too weak or too strong, who have experienced repeated failures with classic IVF, or who have to undergo chemotherapy treatment may also be candidates.

Does Assisted Hatching Improve the Chances of Success?

The purpose of hatching is to help the embryo shed its envelope so it can implant in the uterine wall. It's thought that in some older women this membrane becomes tougher and lowers the probability of embryo implantation. However, little information is available on the impact of this technique on improving birth rates, and it cannot be regularly recommended.

Should Rest Be Prescribed After an Embryo Transfer?

England's National Institute for Health and Care Excellence (NICE) recommends informing patients that resting more than twenty minutes after embryo transfer does not improve success rates. A recent study confirms that remaining in a prone position for thirty minutes after the transfer had no positive effect on IVF success. Studies have even reported a beneficial effect from moderate physical activity following an assisted reproductive technology procedure, with active women having rates of implantation and birth substantially

higher than those who were sedentary. Being immobile or reducing physical activity after IVF should therefore be discouraged; it should instead be suggested to women that they get moderate physical exercise and carry on with their usual daily activities.

Does Having Sexual Relations During the Period of Embryo Transfer Harm the Chances of Conceiving?

Contrary to the fears of many infertile couples, it's clearly established that sexual relations during the period of embryo transfer are not only safe, but might even promote embryo implantation. The mechanisms underlying this improvement in success rates are poorly understood, but it's likely that seminal fluid may induce a favourable immune response in the woman, which heightens the receptivity of the endometrium and promotes embryonic development in the uterus. Sexual relations after embryo transfer should therefore be encouraged, except for women with ovarian hyperstimulation or pelvic pain.

Does Taking Low-Does Aspiring After the Embryo Transfer Improve the Chances of IVF Success?

Low-dose aspirin has been suggested as a way to enhance endometrial receptivity. A detailed analysis of studies has not, however, discerned any improvement in birth rates in women who took aspirin; this drug should not, therefore, be suggested as part of IVF.

What Role Does Acupuncture Play in IVF?

The potentially beneficial role of acupuncture has been seriously assessed in several studies, both during the egg retrieval and

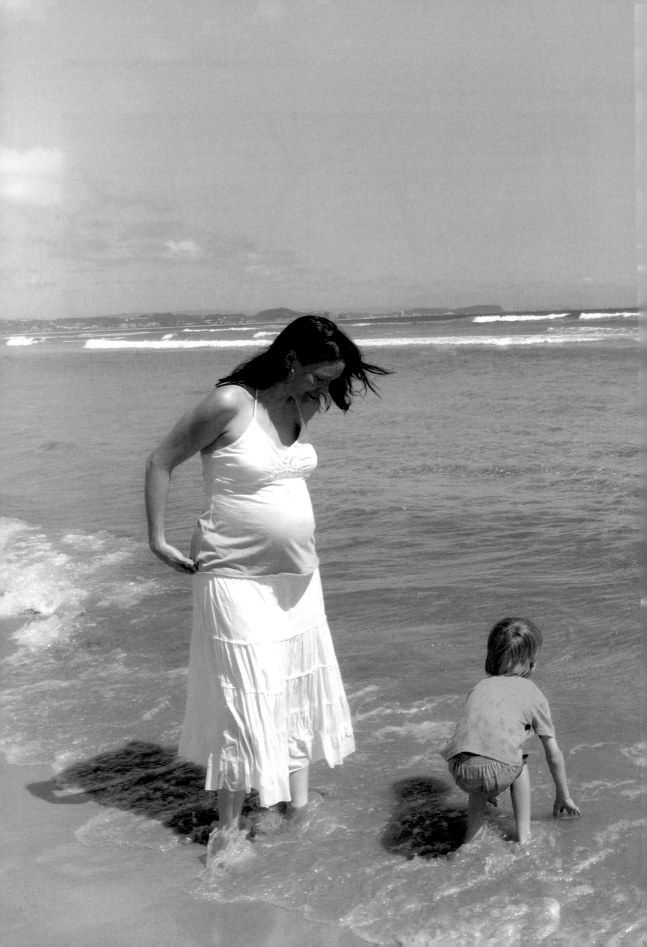

CHAPTER 6

A Legacy of Health

The future is getting ready to be the past
— Pierre Dac (1893–1975)

Pregnancy is an important milestone in a woman's life, an experience of rare intensity involving major changes in her identity, both physical and psychological. Being pregnant is not just carrying an unborn child; it's also having the privilege of experiencing the miracle of life intimately, of being in the front row at the concert of emotions stemming from having a new living being right inside your body. Pregnancy is certainly common and "in the order of things," but it's still one of life's watershed moments, for it's key to achieving what is beyond a doubt the greatest human accomplishment: a child.

Pregnancy is so important that pregnant women often go through it feeling a little anxious and try to do whatever they can so that the child can enjoy the most favourable conditions for its development. And there is no shortage of advice and recommendations! Our intention

here is not to list all of these recommendations, nor to pass judgment on their merits; there's a substantial bibliography devoted to the various stages of pregnancy and, in most cases, these books contain very relevant information that can help couples approach this important event in a calm frame of mind. We believe it useful, however, to review the main principles that should guide every pregnancy, by giving an overview of the major impact the uterine environment has on the child's development, as well as on its future health. Just like our genes, health can also be inherited!

MOTHER-CHILD FUSION

The physiological adaptations that accompany the implanting of the embryo in the uterus are one of the most fascinating aspects of pregnancy. The unborn child is not just present inside its mother's body; it's literally part of her body, drawing from it all of the elements essential to its survival. The placenta is the very embodiment of this fetal-maternal fusion: formed by the union of the mother's endometrium with the layer of cells surrounding the blastocyst (trophoblast), this organ enables maternal blood to reach the fetus and sustain its development by providing it with oxygen and nutrients essential for cell multiplication, while eliminating the waste formed during growth (figure 41). This unique mode of communication, which arose during evolution approximately 170 million years ago, makes the mother-child relationship a highly complex phenomenon, associated with major changes in maternal and fetal physiology.

The most crucial aspect of this relationship remains the fetus's extreme vulnerability, its growth being completely dependent on what it receives through the maternal blood. And this is why pregnancy deserves special attention: by directly affecting the fetus, the mother's lifestyle will have a determining influence not only on its immediate health, but also on its entire life after birth and on that of its descendants. Let's not forget that three generations are simultaneously exposed to the conditions in a pregnant woman's body and environment: her own and that of her child, of course, but also that of her future grandchildren, who will develop from reproductive cells formed during the fetus's development (figure 42). This may be hard to believe at first, but there is a strong likelihood that some of the aspects of your current

UTEROPLACENTAL BLOOD CIRCULATION

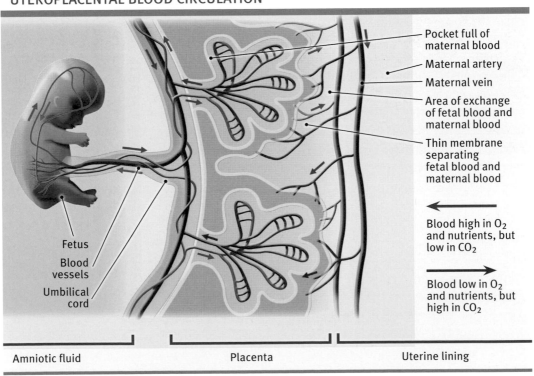

Pocket full of maternal blood

Maternal artery

Maternal vein

Area of exchange of fetal blood and maternal blood

Thin membrane separating fetal blood and maternal blood

← Blood high in O_2 and nutrients, but low in CO_2

→ Blood low in O_2 and nutrients, but high in CO_2

Fetus

Blood vessels

Umbilical cord

Amniotic fluid

Placenta

Uterine lining

FIGURE 41

The Intimate Mother-Child Relationship

In eutherian mammals (having a placenta), the mother's blood communicates directly with fetal circulation to provide oxygen and nutrients essential for fetal development. When we consider the astronomical number of cell divisions required to transform a microscopic embryo, with just a few cells when it implants, into a newborn weighing approximately 3.5 kg made up of many hundreds of billions of cells, we cannot help but be astonished at the efficiency of this system and the beauty and order emerging from such complexity.

The close contact between mother and child obviously has major repercussions on the physiology of both partners in this "blood link." For example, throughout its development, the fetus expresses an equal mixture of proteins from the mother and father on the surface of its cells. Immunologically speaking, this situation is extremely unusual, since the father's antigens should be detected by the mother's immune system as the signal of an "intruder" inside the body, a bit like what happens with an organ transplant. How the immune system manages to give special status to the fetus remains one of the great mysteries of biology, but it seems that certain T lymphocytes (white cells) are able to reduce the immune response to the fetus by accumulating in large numbers in the placenta. The importance of these regulating lymphocytes is clearly seen when there are serious complications during pregnancy, notably preeclampsia, correlated with the abnormal development of these lymphocytes.

Mother-child communication is not, however, one way; several studies indicate that cells from the fetus migrate into the mother's body and can be detected in her blood and bones several decades after the pregnancy. The impact of this phenomenon, called microchimerism, is still not understood, but some think that these undifferentiated embryonic cells could play a role in repairing damaged tissues. Interestingly, a recent study showed that the presence of fetal cells in the mother's brain was associated with a decreased risk of Alzheimer's disease.

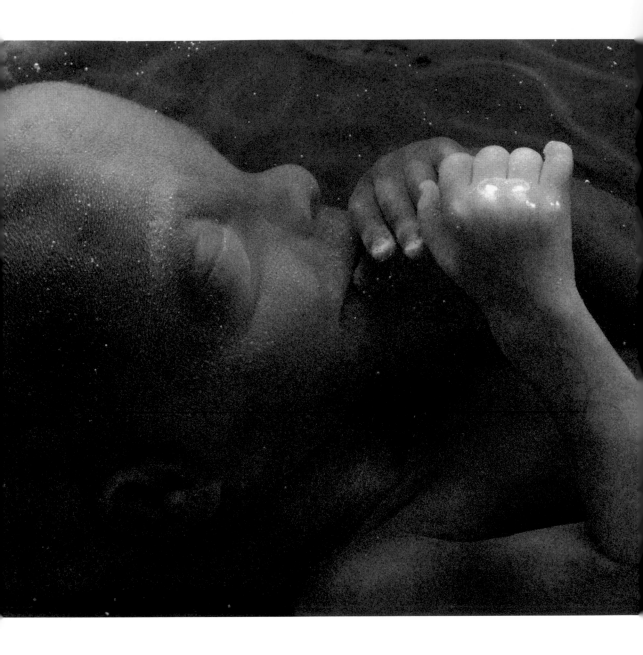

health are a direct consequence of the way your grandparents lived! Pregnancy is therefore one of the most important phases of life, not only because it's essential for the development of the fetus, but also because of its long-term influence on the health and overall wellbeing of the child, even when he or she reaches adulthood.

SUPPORTING A COMPLEX PROCESS

The creation of a human being during pregnancy is in a way a condensed version of evolution, the completion in just nine months of a series of molecular events that have occurred little by little during the four billion years of life on Earth. The embryonic development of our skeleton, our nervous system, and our organs does not happen by chance; each of these stages has been optimized over millions of years, gradually improving because of the selection of the genes that best enabled people to adapt to the difficulties imposed by the environment. This gradual evolution is clearly illustrated in the striking resemblance of the early stages of the human embryo to those of animal species as distant from each other as trout, turtles, or chickens (figure 43). We need to remember, therefore, that we are the heirs to a long process of selection, and that it's only because of the expression of genes selected in the course of evolution that human complexity can be expressed during fetal development. The goal of pregnancy is thus to do everything possible to create a favourable climate for the expression of these genes, to give them the tools they need to perform well and enable the fetus to reach its full human potential.

EATING WELL

In addition to being very important for fertility, a pregnant woman's diet is the factor with the most influence on fetal development. The first reflex is often to approach these new nutritional requirements from the perspective of quantity, to "eat for two," as is often said, so that the fetus doesn't lack for anything. While this is a normal attitude, it's important to understand that the energy needs of a developing fetus are quite low, especially during the first trimester of pregnancy: in general, a caloric increase of barely 10 to 15 percent (or about 200 calories, the equivalent of three apples or a portion of nuts) is more than enough

to maintain fetal development. The essential nutrients (vitamins, minerals, proteins, fats) are needed mainly for embryonic cell multiplication and the development of all of the structures that enable the child to be born in good health (figure 44). Although in our era of dietary abundance it's easy (and tempting!) to nibble on anything and everything to get the extra calories needed, what's actually important is to try to eat "twice as well," so that the extra food eaten will first and foremost go to providing the

THE ENVIRONMENTAL CONDITIONS A PREGNANT WOMAN IS EXPOSED TO HAVE AN IMPACT ON THREE GENERATIONS

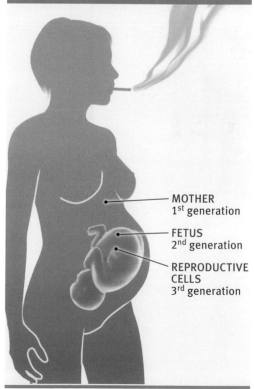

MOTHER
1st generation

FETUS
2nd generation

REPRODUCTIVE CELLS
3rd generation

FIGURE 42

elements indispensable for fetal growth, as well as supporting the physiological changes taking place in the mother's body.

In our daily lives, it's usually very difficult, not to say impossible, to determine precisely the calorie and nutrient content of what we eat. However, it's possible to deal with this problem by following three simple rules.

1. Eat lots of plant foods (fruits, vegetables, pulses, etc.) and avoid foods that are high in calories but low in nutrients (chips, candies, soft drinks, junk food in general). In this way, the additional food intake will automatically equal an increase in nutrients essential to fetal growth.

2. For pregnant women who do not eat properly, for example because of nausea, taking vitamin supplements can prevent malnutrition and ensure an adequate intake of essential vitamins and minerals. Note that even when there are no health problems, most doctors recommend taking these supplements, given the low proportion of the population (25 percent) who eat the recommended quantities of plant foods.

THE EMBRYOS OF VARIOUS VERTEBRATES, IN DIFFERENT STAGES OF DEVELOPMENT

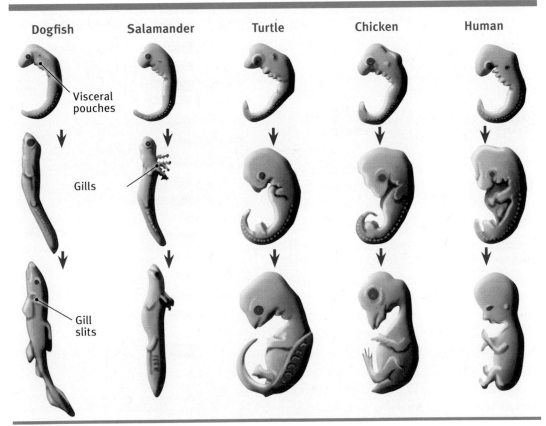

FIGURE 43

3. The easiest way to determine whether caloric intake is sufficient is to measure weight gain during pregnancy. On average, 25 percent of the kilos put on during pregnancy are due to the baby's weight, 50 percent to the physiological changes that are part of its development (blood volume, uterus, placenta, etc.), and the last quarter is an energy reserve (figure 46). For women with a normal weight at the beginning of the pregnancy (BMI around 25), a gain of 11 to 16 kilos is usually recommended; however, women who are overweight at the beginning (and who therefore already have extra energy stored) should limit this gain, especially if they are obese (figure 45). The ideal diet for a pregnant woman is not that complicated; it's essentially a matter of getting most of her calories from healthy foods, for example plants high in essential nutrients, while avoiding as much as possible foods full of empty calories that provide too much energy and, at the same time, lack nutrients useful for fetal development. But in addition to these main principles, at least two specific points must also be considered.

Sufficient Folate Intake

Folate is a B vitamin (B9) that plays a key role in the multiplication of embryonic cells. This vitamin is especially important during the first month of fetal growth, when the neural tube that ultimately becomes the child's nervous system is formed. The embryonic cells in this region divide at a frantic pace during this period (their population doubles every five hours approximately); they therefore need very high folate intake to sustain this growth, five to ten

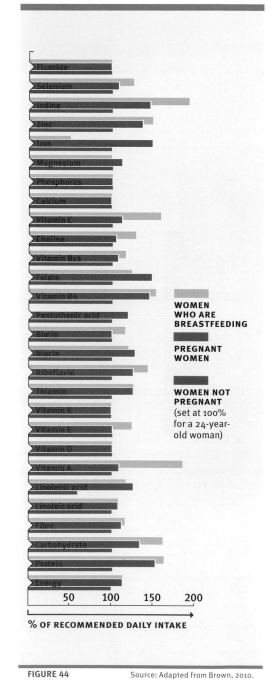

NUTRIENT REQUIREMENTS: WOMEN WHO ARE BREASTFEEDING, PREGNANT WOMEN, WOMEN NOT PREGNANT

% OF RECOMMENDED DAILY INTAKE

FIGURE 44 Source: Adapted from Brown, 2010.

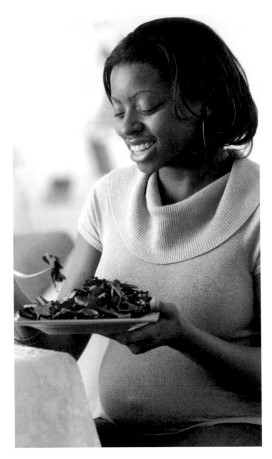

RECOMMENDED WEIGHT GAIN DURING PREGNANCY ACCORDING TO THE MOTHER'S BODY MASS INDEX AT TIME OF CONCEPTION

Weight category	Total weight gain	
	KILOGRAMS	POUNDS
UNDERWEIGHT (BMI ‹ 18.5)	13 to 18	28 to 40
NORMAL WEIGHT (BMI of 18.5 to 24.9)	11 to 16	25 to 35
OVERWEIGHT (BMI of 25 to 29.9)	7 to 11	15 to 25
OBESE (BMI ≥ 30)	5 to 9	11 to 20

FIGURE 45   Source: Adapted from Brown, 2010.

times more than in a woman who is not pregnant. Folate is found in considerable amounts in several fruits and vegetables (spinach, asparagus, broccoli, oranges) and foods made from fortified flour (cereals, pasta), but the easiest way to ensure that the fetus receives the required amounts of this vitamin is still to take a daily dose of supplements with a minimum of 0.4 mg of folic acid (the synthetic form of folate). For women not at personal risk, this can be in the form of a multivitamin supplement containing folic acid (0.4 to 1 mg), beginning at least three months before conception and continuing throughout the pregnancy and the post-partum period (4 to 6 weeks), as long as the woman is breastfeeding.

For some patients who are considered at higher risk because of various health problems (epilepsy, insulin-dependent diabetes, obesity, a family history of neural tube abnormalities, belonging to certain ethnic groups, Sikhs, for example), increased dietary intake of folate-rich foods and multivitamins containing 5 mg folic acid is recommended. The increased folic acid supplementation starts at least three months before conception and continues until the tenth or twelfth week after conception. It's then replaced by the more standard multivitamin supplement, containing 0.4 to 1 mg of folic acid.

Sufficient folate intake is critical to prevent neural tube abnormalities like spina bifida (protrusion of the spinal cord outside the spine) and anencephaly (absence of a brain). Anencephalic children die in the uterus or shortly after birth, while those with spina bifida survive, but often have significant physical handicaps. In addition to preventing

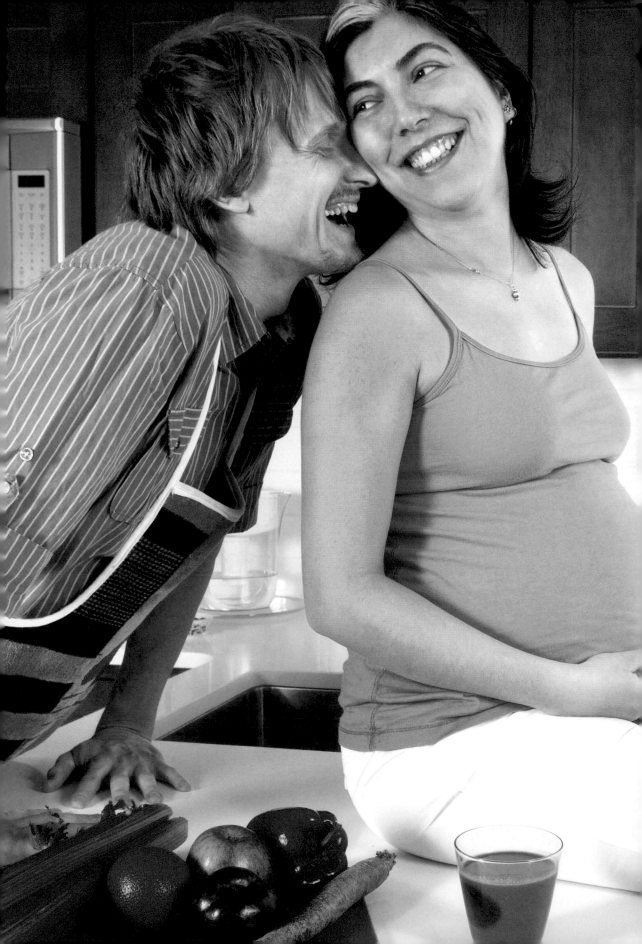

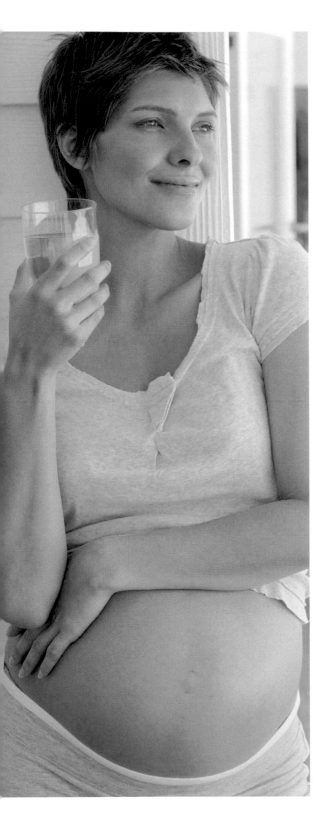

these abnormalities, a recent study suggests that a high intake of folic acid (0.6 mg per day) during the first trimester of pregnancy is associated with a considerable decrease (40 percent) in the risk of autism. However, it's important to note that neural tube abnormalities appear very early in fetal development, between the third and fourth week of pregnancy, at a time when women very often don't know they're pregnant. When the pregnancy is planned, the risk of abnormalities can be significantly reduced by taking folic acid supplements as soon as contraception is stopped or even a few months before; otherwise, a diet high in folic acid can play an extremely important role in preventing these abnormalities.

Omega-3 Fatty Acids

Omega-3s are essential fats we can't produce ourselves and which must therefore come from our diet. There are two main types of omega-3s: short-chain omega-3s in plants, mainly flax seeds and some nuts (especially walnuts), and long-chain omega-3s from animal sources, found almost exclusively in fatty fish and some sea algae. Many studies have shown that long-chain omega-3s play many positive roles in the proper functioning of our bodies and are absolutely essential for the development of brain and retina cells during pregnancy. Unfortunately, the modern western diet is seriously deficient in omega-3 fatty acids and most pregnant women have blood concentrations of docosahexaenoic acid (DHA) and eicosapentaenoic acid (EPA) below recommended levels. A recent study indicates, however, that this deficiency can easily be corrected by simply eating two servings of salmon a week.

AVERAGE DISTRIBUTION OF WEIGHT GAINED DURING PREGNANCY

Weight		Distribution
KILOS	**POUNDS**	
3.4	7.5	Average baby's weight
3.2	7	Extra stored protein, fats, and other nutrients
1.8	4	Extra blood
1.8	4	Other additional body fluids
0.9	2	Breast enlargement
0.9	2	Uterine enlargement
0.9	2	Amniotic fluids
0.7	1.5	Placenta

FIGURE 46   Source: Adapted from Brown, 2010.

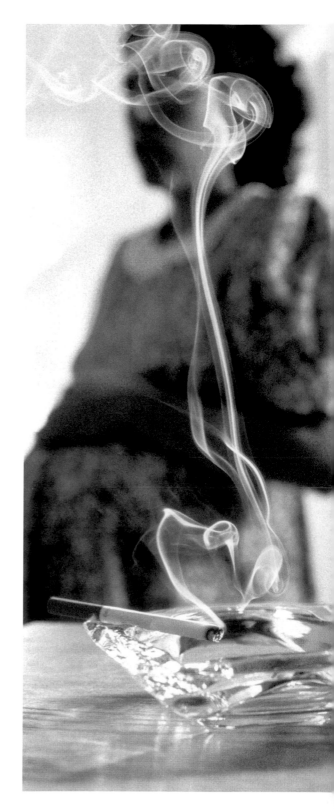

AVOIDING TOXIC SUBSTANCES

In addition to having to rely on an optimal intake of essential nutrients, fetal development must also be able to occur in a healthy environment, free of toxic substances that can disrupt the mechanisms involved in the multiplication and specialization of fetal cells. While we can't eradicate all of the contaminants that are part of the world we live in, it's nonetheless possible to limit the damage done by some of them.

Tobacco
Smoking alone is thought to be responsible for 20 to 30 percent of low birth weight babies, with low birth weight being

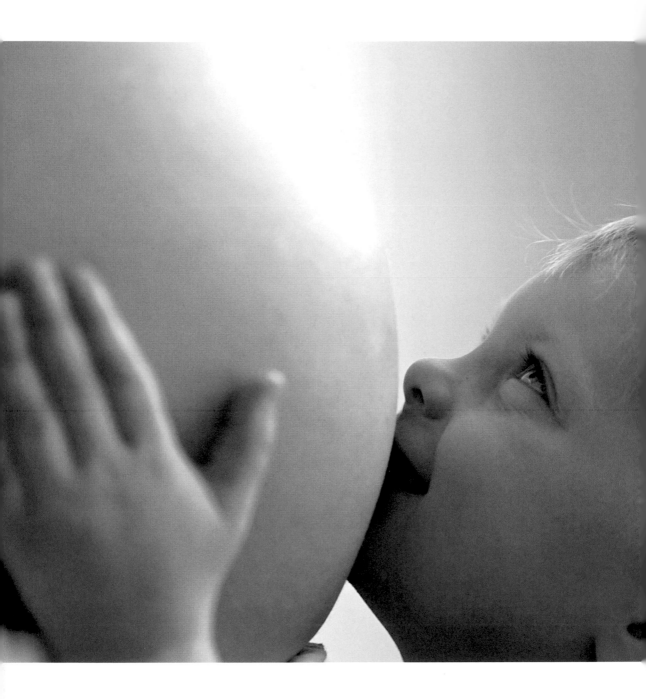

one of the main risk factors for chronic diseases in adulthood (see later in the text). Pregnant women who smoke are also at a higher risk of giving birth to a child with defective cardiovascular, respiratory, and musculoskeletal systems. Children of mothers who smoked during pregnancy are also more likely to have behavioural problems, attention deficit disorders, and poor academic achievement. Yet while women know about these catastrophic effects both on their health and on their child's health, just half of women smokers succeed in not smoking during pregnancy; nicotine is a highly addictive substance and some people have structural variations in the receptors for this drug that make them especially sensitive to its effects. There's no miracle solution to stop smoking, but there do exist a number of tools to help women smokers who want to quit: nicotine substitutes, support groups, websites dedicated to fighting smoking, or even taking up interesting activities. The best source of motivation, however, is still to tell oneself that quitting smoking is, by far, the action that will have the most positive repercussions on the child's life, in both the short and long term.

Alcohol

Alcohol is a substance that very easily passes through the placenta and interferes with developing organs, since the fetus's liver is immature and cannot detoxify the alcohol as effectively as in adulthood. In large doses, there is a risk of causing fetal alcohol syndrome, which affects approximately three children out of every thousand and is characterized by overall stunted growth, several physical abnormalities, and significant brain damage leading to serious developmental delays and learning difficulties. In North America, fetal alcohol syndrome is one of the main causes of cognitive impairment, on a par with trisomy 21 (Down syndrome).

In practice, the minimum amount of alcohol that could be consumed during pregnancy is not known. Most studies carried out to date indicate that having more than one drink a day has a negative impact on the fetal nervous system; however, harmful

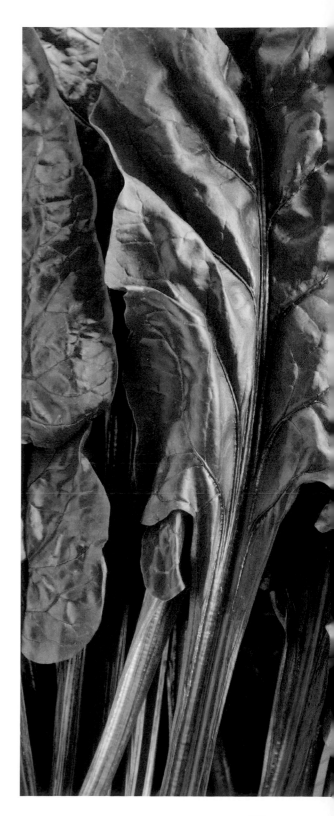

effects have also been reported for much lower doses, and as a result it is possible that alcohol causes some damage, even in tiny amounts. As with tobacco, abstinence from alcohol is really the only option for pregnant women who are trying to optimize their future child's development.

Dietary Toxins

During pregnancy, the effectiveness of a woman's immune system is slightly reduced so that the body can tolerate the fetus. The negative side of this adaptation is that the future mother is less able to fight infections; this is why pregnant women are usually advised to refrain from eating foods more likely to contain pathogens, especially raw meat or fish, raw milk cheese, and unpasteurized juices. These pathogens can sometimes have a violent impact; the listeriosis agent (Listeria monocytogenes), in particular, can cause premature birth and even, in some cases, fetal death. However, it isn't just germs in food we have to be wary of: substances added as preservatives can also have harmful effects on fetal health. For example, nitrites and nitrates, found in large amounts in a great many processed meat products, are metabolized into nitrosamines that attach themselves to the DNA and can cause mutations that increase the risk of cancer. Studies have reported that children of women who ate significant amounts of foods containing these preservatives during pregnancy had a higher risk of brain tumours.

PROGRAMMING THE FETUS

In addition to having an effect on the short-term health of the fetus, a pregnant woman's lifestyle has an impact on the risk of chronic diseases that can affect the child in the longer term, when he or she reaches adulthood. A striking example of this was the Dutch hongerwinter famine ("the winter of hunger" in Dutch) that occurred at the end of the Second World War. From November 1944 to February 1945, a drastic lack of food forced more than four million Dutch to make do with a calorie intake of fewer than one thousand calories per day, and sometimes much less in certain parts of the country. For women who were pregnant during this period, this serious food deficiency obviously had noticeable impacts on their babies' development, one of which was a lower birth weight. When the fetus has to deal with food shortage during its intrauterine development, it adapts to the nutrient deficiency by focussing on the formation of certain essential organs like the brain, usually to the detriment of the skeleton and the lower limbs. However, later studies showed that these children were at higher risk of becoming obese in adulthood and had a cardiovascular disease-related mortality rate much higher than their compatriots whose mothers had not lived through the great famine. How can a paradox like this be explained?

We now know that a fetus can be "programmed" by its mother's living conditions; in other words, the expression of certain genes involved in metabolism is modulated by the information the fetus receives during its development. In famine conditions, the Dutch children acquired during their development the ability to grow in a world where food was scarce and, as a result, preferentially expressed certain genes that enabled them to store food energy more efficiently. However, if

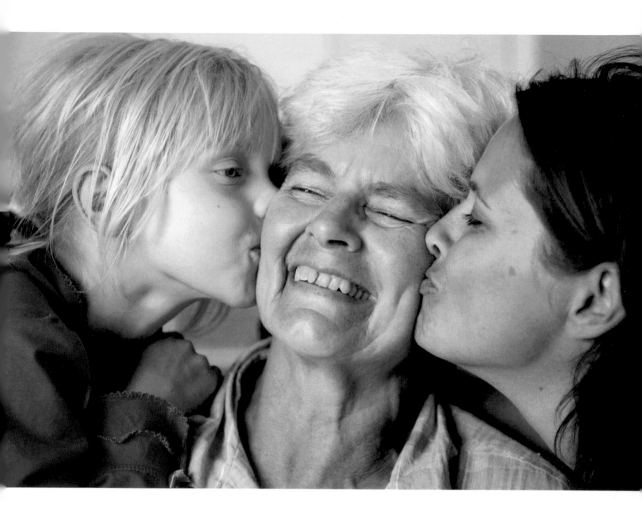

external conditions change after birth, as was the case in Holland with the return to a plentiful food supply at the end of the war, this adaptation becomes a double-edged sword: the heightened ability to extract energy from food can cause a very fast "catching up" and excessive weight gain, at the same time increasing the risk of obesity and diseases associated with being overweight (heart disease, Type 2 diabetes). This concept of "fetal origins of adult disease" implies, therefore, that the fetus is not just a simple "passenger" growing passively in the mother's belly; on the contrary, it's very receptive to everything happening in the environment, almost as if it can accurately "read" the conditions it will have to deal with once it's born and tries to adapt immediately to improve its chances of survival.

INTERGENERATIONAL HEALTH

We have long known that heredity is a complex phenomenon, a mixture of genetic baggage and the cultural context in which a person develops. For example, identical twins, with exactly the same genes, will develop completely different personalities, interests, and abilities as they grow up,

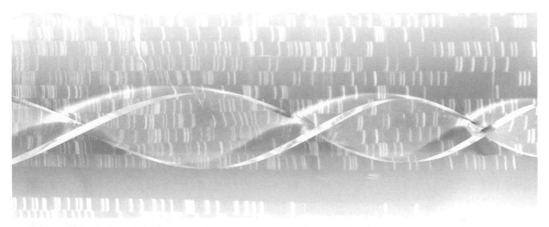

Genomic Imprints

DNA is an extremely stable structure, which changes only very slowly over time. For example, around five thousand years ago a mutation enabling adults to digest milk appeared in pastoral societies, and it's estimated that it took roughly another one thousand years for this mutation to become widespread in those populations (even today, 75 percent of human beings do not have this mutation). The relative inertia of the genome works fine for long-term adaptations, but makes any rapid response to sudden change impossible. To get around this limitation, nature has given cells a rapid reaction mechanism, in which signals from the environment act as interrupters to activate or inhibit the expression of genes in our DNA. For example, adding or removing certain chemical groups in DNA can modify its degree of compaction and thus the expression of certain genes can be facilitated or suppressed: when DNA is decondensed, there is enough space for gene transcription; conversely, with tightly bound DNA, this expression is inhibited. Because of this unusually elegant mechanism, events that affect parents can be communicated to subsequent generations very quickly, without requiring any mutation in the DNA sequence.

As mentioned in the main text, certain lifestyle factors, especially chronic stress and dietary make-up, are known to influence the fetus via epigenetics. Mothers subjected to intense stress, for example, have very high cortisol levels (the stress hormone) that reach the fetus through the placenta. This abnormal increase in cortisol has a negative effect on gene expression in the hypothalamic-pituitary-adrenal axis involved in the stress response and is associated with lower birth weight and an increase in blood pressure in adulthood, as well as a higher risk of anxiety disorders.

especially if they are separated shortly after birth. This cooperation between nature and culture is in a way the signature of human identity, with the result that each of us acquires a unique personality, reflecting the influence of our social environment and the interests and aptitudes we develop over time.

The fetus's remarkable malleability in response to its mother's lifestyle indicates that the gestation period is another factor in defining a person's identity. Strictly speaking, this influence is neither genetic nor cultural, but instead epigenetic, meaning that it combines both of these elements, with environmental factors

FACTORS THAT CAN CAUSE FETAL EPIGENETIC MODIFICATIONS

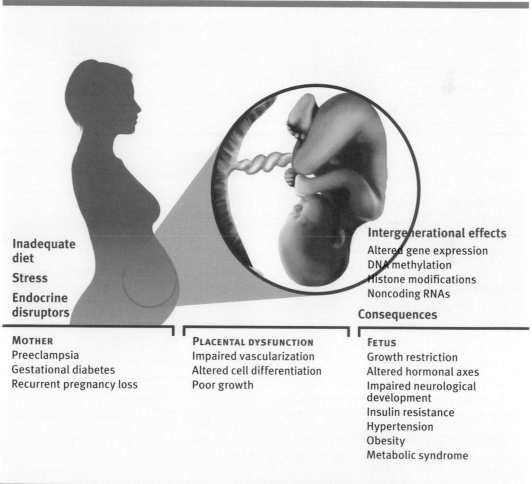

Inadequate diet

Stress

Endocrine disruptors

Intergenerational effects
Altered gene expression
DNA methylation
Histone modifications
Noncoding RNAs

Consequences

MOTHER	PLACENTAL DYSFUNCTION	FETUS
Preeclampsia	Impaired vascularization	Growth restriction
Gestational diabetes	Altered cell differentiation	Altered hormonal axes
Recurrent pregnancy loss	Poor growth	Impaired neurological development
		Insulin resistance
		Hypertension
		Obesity
		Metabolic syndrome

FIGURE 47

subtly modulating the expression of certain genes to improve adaptation to these conditions (see box). This is why the maternal lifestyle has such an impact on the child's long-term health: by introducing modifications to the genetic baggage of the fetus during its development, the mother leaves an indelible imprint that will have a lifelong influence on the child.

Epigenetic modifications often have harmful repercussions when they occur in response to "attacks" on the fetus during its development. Malnutrition is not the only one that can change the fetus's genetic baggage: several factors linked to lifestyle, like chronic stress, smoking, and alcohol consumption, as well as some placental circulation disorders, also cause epigenetic modifications, with long-term consequences for the child's health (figure 47). In most cases, these "attacks" on the fetus hinder its development and are associated with lower birth weight, as well as impairing metabolism and the development of certain organs (pancreas, kidneys, fatty tissues). In addition to increasing the risk of certain chronic diseases, hypertension, for example, these developmental abnormalities often result in hormonal imbalances that profoundly disrupt metabolism and can result in the development of obesity and Type 2 diabetes. These problems are especially obvious when there is a notable discrepancy between conditions in the intrauterine environment and those in which the child grows up; for example, a person born in a poor country who emigrates to a country where food is abundant, or one who lives in a country in economic transition and adopts western food habits (especially junk food), are both exposed to a calorie intake that is at

PERCENTAGE OF CHILDREN BORN IN CANADA BETWEEN 1984 AND 2010 WEIGHING LESS THAN 2.5 KG AT BIRTH

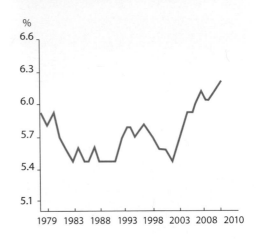

FIGURE 48   Source: Statistics Canada, 2012.

LOW BIRTH WEIGHT: SOME CONSEQUENCES FOR ADULT HEALTH

- Hypertension
- Type 2 diabetes
- Obesity, metabolic syndrome
- Coronary disease
- Stroke
- Osteoporosis
- Depression and psychoses (for example, schizophrenia)
- Cognitive losses due to aging
- Chronic renal failure
- Impaired gonadic reaction that can lead to disease
- Impaired auto-immune reaction that can lead to disease
- Lower life expectancy

FIGURE 49

odds with the conditions of scarcity they developed in during the fetal period and are, as a result, at much higher risk of developing one or another of these diseases.

However, it would be wrong to believe that this is a problem exclusive to poor countries or those in economic transition: in most developed countries, including Canada, the proportion of low birth weight babies (under 2.5 kg) has increased in recent decades and currently makes up more than 6 percent of births (figure 48). Since low birth weight is a major risk factor for later chronic diseases (figure 49), especially cardiovascular disease and Type 2 diabetes, pregnant women would do well to adopt a lifestyle that promotes optimal fetal development so the child can be born and grow up in good health.

While nutritional deficiencies and exposure to toxins like tobacco and alcohol can be damaging to the fetus, this does not mean it's necessary to go to the other extreme by providing it with too many calories. As they say, "Too much is as bad as too little." In fact, several studies have clearly shown that too much food can also create "fetal stress," with a negative effect on the child's development and adult health. For example, blood sugar and insulin levels that are too high, as a result of overeating and obesity, can leave a "metabolic imprint" on a fetus developing in these abnormal conditions. To deal with the extra sugar in the maternal blood reaching it through the placenta, the fetal pancreas has to secrete large quantities of insulin, and this early hyperinsulinemia

INTERGENERATIONAL PATHWAYS AND FETAL PROGRAMMING

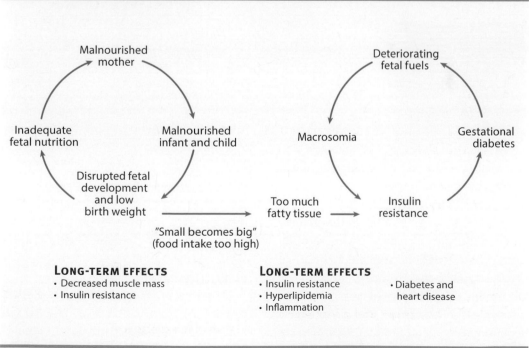

FIGURE 50

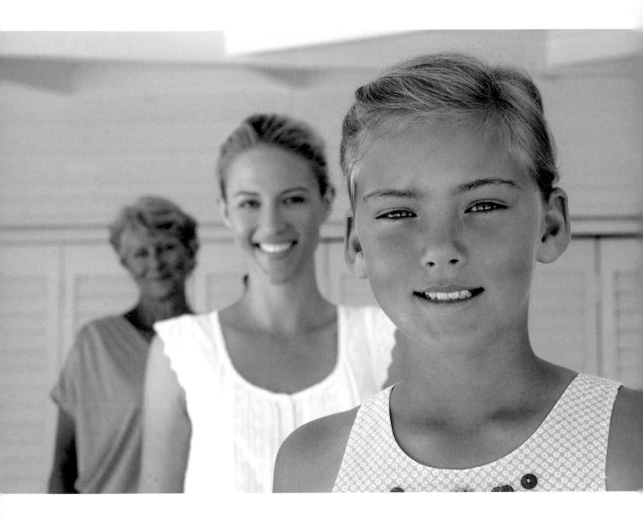

considerably increases the risk of obesity and diabetes in adulthood.

Metabolic and hormonal imbalances associated with obesity and maternal diabetes also affect the development of the neuronal circuits involved in appetite control and the feeling of fullness, which predisposes the fetus to develop dietary and metabolic disorders during its lifetime. These metabolic imprints bequeathed by the mother can also occur even in the absence of obesity or diabetes: for example, a recent study has shown that women with a poor quality diet (too much saturated fat, lack of fibre and essential nutrients) are at

greater risk of having elevated blood sugar and insulin levels and, as a result, of giving birth to babies who already have a diabetogenic profile at birth. What's more, the fetus may develop an attraction to these surplus energy sources: according to recent research, the brains of children of mothers who ate large quantities of junk food have a higher "tolerance" to these foods and these children may therefore need to eat more of them to feel satisfied.

In several respects, obesity and being overweight can be as harmful to the child's health as nutritional deficiencies, not to mention that this excess weight significantly increases the risk of a number of complications during pregnancy (especially hypertension and gestational diabetes) and during delivery (cesareans, postpartum bleeding). For women who want to have a child, a healthy diet and maintaining a normal body weight before and during pregnancy must be objectives of primary importance.

While the influence of maternal diet on the health of the unborn child is intuitively easy to understand, recent studies suggest that the father's type of diet could also have repercussions for the newborn. It has recently been observed that daughters whose father had a diet high in fat quickly showed an intolerance to sugar, as well as a loss of their ability to secrete insulin. These abnormalities are associated with major changes in the expression profile of several genes in the pancreatic cells. Similarly, children whose fathers had a protein-deficient diet showed abnormalities in the expression of several genes involved in the metabolism of fats and cholesterol. Therefore, men may also therefore play an important role in the health of their offspring by adopting healthy food habits.

INFLUENCING OUR GRANDCHILDREN

As was mentioned earlier, the conditions in which pregnancy occurs do not simply influence the health of the fetus, but also that of its offspring. Epigenetic modifications brought about by too little or too much food, stress, or toxins like tobacco can, in fact, affect the fetus's reproductive cells and thus be incorporated into the genetic baggage of its offspring several decades later. Children's health is therefore not just a question of "good genes"; it also depends on the various environments these genes have been exposed to during the gestation period. For example, a daughter with too low a birth weight has a higher risk of becoming obese in adulthood, owing to metabolic damage during the fetal period. When she, in turn, gets pregnant, this excess weight will trigger the onset of metabolic disorders like insulin resistance and hyperglycemia, which will program the fetal metabolism and predispose it to developing various metabolic diseases in adulthood (figure 50). The nutritional deficiency experienced by the grandmother during her pregnancy is thus largely responsible for her granddaughter's health problems! This intergenerational epigenetic transmission helps to explain why members of some families, or economically disadvantaged classes, have a tendency not to live as long, even in the absence of genes that predispose them to developing serious diseases like cancer or heart disease. Luckily, epigenetic modifications are reversible and it's possible to put an end to these cycles of metabolic imbalances by adopting a healthy lifestyle during pregnancy, and creating a fetal environment free of toxic substances that lets the fetus know it is in an environment where food is neither scarce nor too plentiful. While in psychology it's said that everything is decided before age four, it could also be said that much of a person's health is determined even before birth!

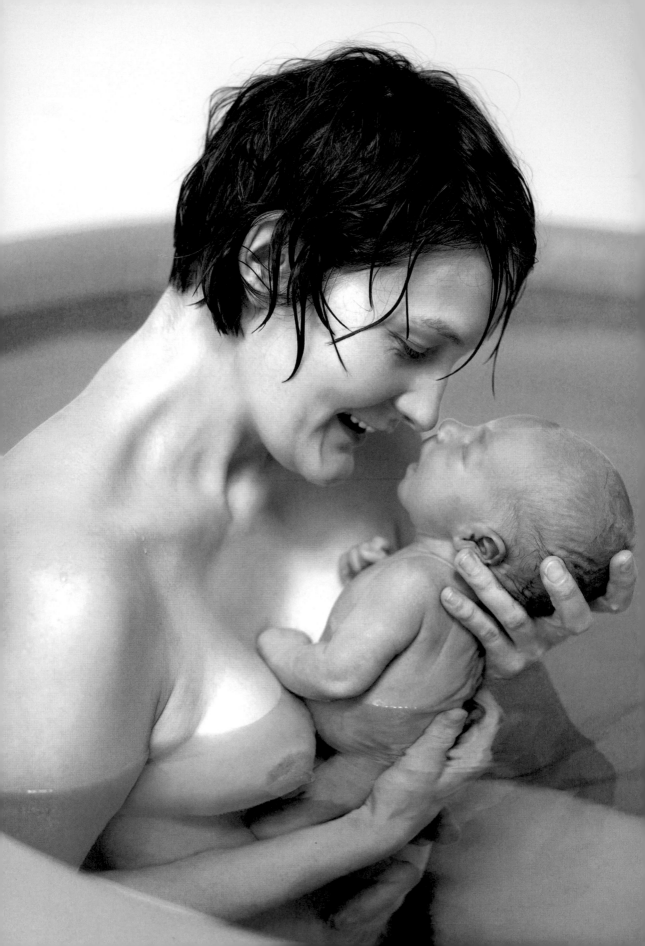

CHAPTER 7

Screening and Prenatal Diagnosis

On large boats without sails
I already see you climbing on board
Among the stars
You'll sail
My child my brother
Among the stars
You'll sail
— GILLES VIGNEAULT (1928–)

One of the most fascinating aspects of embryonic development is that a fertilized egg can, by itself, generate a human being made up of several hundreds of billions of distinct cells. This incredibly complex process has hardly given up all of its secrets, but we know that it depends on the genetic information contained in the maternal and paternal chromosomes, with the roughly 20,000 to 30,000 genes on these chromosomes precisely coordinating the sequence of events that will ultimately lead to the creation of a new life. To develop properly, the fetus has to be able to count on both the integrity of the fertilized egg's genetic material and on the control of this genetic activity as the various body structures are being formed.

Such a complex process is obviously not perfect: chance alone makes it inevitable that errors happen at one or another of the many stages required for the embryo to develop normally and cause sometimes serious fetal abnormalities. As a result, a challenge of modern medicine is to identify these abnormalities as early as possible so that parents can quickly be reassured about their child's health or, if the news is not good, can have in hand all of the information necessary to decide on the pregnancy's outcome.

SCREENING OR PRENATAL DIAGNOSIS?

While chance is an intrinsic part of life, it's in our nature to try to anticipate events that will happen in the future. Pregnancy is one of the best examples of this quest for an answer in the face of an uncertain future: in every era, women have wanted to find out quickly whether they were carrying a child, wanted or not, and this curiosity led very early on to the development of reliable pregnancy tests (see page 143). Owing to medical progress, we can now go one step further and not only confirm the existence of a fetus in the early stages of pregnancy, but also determine whether it's healthy and identify the risk of abnormalities that may jeopardize its health.

Prenatal screening as we know it today has its origins in prenatal diagnosis, which developed with amniocentesis. First of all, it's important to distinguish between the terms "screening" and "diagnosis": prenatal screening is a non-intrusive medical examination requiring only interventions that are harmless for the fetus, like a fetal ultrasound, with or without a blood test from the mother-to-be. By integrating all the data obtained during a screening examination, a statistical assessment of risk can be established — the probability that the fetus has or does not have a serious abnormality. While screening never offers an absolute guarantee as to the fetus's health, most often it proves to be reassuring.

To obtain a definitive answer, as to the number of chromosomes in the fetal cells, for example, prenatal diagnosis is required. Two intrusive techniques are currently used, amniocentesis, which involves withdrawing amniotic fluid containing fetal cells, using a needle, or trophoblast biopsy (choriocentesis), in which placental cells (placental villi), which indirectly reflect the composition of fetal chromosomes, are sampled. In both cases, a detailed analysis of the chromosomes inside these cells usually makes it possible to arrive at a firm diagnosis.

Because they are intrusive, prenatal diagnostic methods always carry a degree of risk of pregnancy loss (1 percent of cases). Minimizing this risk is why prenatal screening was developed: by making it possible to establish with a high level of confidence the likelihood that a fetus is normal, screening can reduce the number of risky diagnostic procedures and save them for women who are really at highest risk.

EARLY PRENATAL SCREENING BETWEEN THE ELEVENTH AND FOURTEENTH WEEKS

Several developmental abnormalities can already be detected very early on by doing prenatal screening between the eleventh and fourteenth weeks of pregnancy.

CHROMOSOMAL ABNORMALITIES IN NUMBER (ANEUPLOIDIES)

During fertilization, the twenty-three chromosomes in the head of the sperm cell merge with the twenty-three chromosomes in the egg to form a "diploid" cell, possessing two copies of each chromosome. However, defects sometimes occur when reproductive cells are being created, and the egg or sperm may contain an extra copy of a given chromosome; if one or the other of these cells participates in fertilization, the embryo will contain, right from the start, one chromosome too many. The ploidy of these cells is therefore "not good" and they are called "aneuploidies" (from the Greek *aneu*, meaning "not good"). In most cases, aneuploidy makes fetal development impossible and results in a spontaneous abortion before the tenth week of pregnancy (50 percent of pregnancy losses are caused by chromosomal abnormalities). On the other hand, some aneuploidies

Nefertiti's Pregnancy Test

↗ Medical papyrus dating from the eighteenth dynasty (c. 1500 BCE), similar to the Berlin papyrus.

Universally recognized for the architectural genius of its monuments, the Egypt of the pharaohs was also very advanced in medical knowledge. According to a papyrus dating from the Middle Empire (2033 to 1786 BCE), it was common practice for the women of ancient Egypt to pour a few drops of their urine onto a sample of barley and emmer (a type of wheat), each in a canvas bag, every day. If the barley and wheat both germinated after a few days, it meant that the woman was pregnant and would give birth. We may smile at this kind of practice, but it's nonetheless true that the Egyptians had actually developed the first pregnancy test in the history of humanity. In 1963, a rigorous scientific analysis showed that in 70 percent of cases urine from pregnant women stimulated grain germination, whereas that of non-pregnant women had no effect. It appears that the higher amounts of hormones during pregnancy mimic the action of plant growth hormones and promote the plant's growth.

are viable, but have serious physiological repercussions for the child; as a result, identifying these abnormalities provides critical information to guide parents in their decision as to whether or not to continue with an abnormal pregnancy.

Trisomy 21

Caused by an extra 21st chromosome, this trisomy is the most common and best-described viable chromosomal abnormality. It occurs in approximately one out of every seven hundred births and its incidence increases considerably with parental age, especially that of the mother (figure 52). Whereas at age 25 a woman has a risk of 1 in 1,380 of being pregnant with a trisomic child, this risk can rise to 1 in 43 by age 45. These children are recognizable by their unusual features (flat face, flat nose, short neck, round ears, etc.); they have various degrees of mental delay and many physical defects (cardiac, intestinal, anal imperforation, etc.).

Trisomy 18

Also known as Edwards syndrome, this trisomy is the second most frequently diagnosed chromosomal aberration, occurring in approximately 1 out of 7,000 cases. For the vast majority (95 percent), this condition causes death in utero. For a reason still poorly understood, the survival rate for female fetuses is higher, which explains the preponderance of girls with trisomy 18 at birth. The possession of an extra 18th chromosome is accompanied by several physical defects and significant mental delay. Nearly 90 percent of children with this syndrome will die before they are a year old. At the present time, medical treatment for children with this disease is limited to care and comfort only, as even

surgical treatments to correct the physical defects do not alter the natural course of the disease very much.

Trisomy 13

This trisomy, also known as Patau syndrome, causes abnormalities in many organs. This is one of the rarest chromosomal abnormalities in number, with an incidence estimated at approximately 1 case out of every 10,000. Although most fetuses with trisomy 13 die during pregnancy, a small proportion of them are born and will be seriously handicapped. Nearly 80 percent of those born with trisomy 13 will die as a result of their handicaps during the first month of life and only 5 percent will reach the age of three. These children suffer especially from serious psychomotor delays, have convulsions, and experience difficulties in eating normally.

More than 90 percent of the major aneuploidies like trisomies 21, 18, and 13 can be detected between the eleventh and fourteenth weeks of pregnancy, by a combination of fetal nuchal translucency (accumulation of fluid under the skin of the fetus's neck, visible with ultrasound) (see photos) and the level in the mother's blood of two proteins originating from the placenta, the unbound fraction of βhCG and Protein A associated with pregnancy (PAPP-A). This prenatal aneuploidy screening test can be taken even further by testing a sample of the mother's blood earlier, around the ninth or tenth week, followed by fetal ultrasound at twelve weeks, or by adding in other ultrasound assessments of the nasal bone and measurements of blood flows in the ductus venosus (extension of the umbilical vein in the abdomen) and in the fetal tricuspid valve. By combining

PRENATAL SCREENING

 = NORMAL   = ABNORMAL

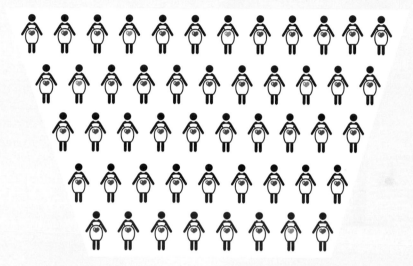

SCREENING
Non-invasive technique
Low-cost technique
Estimation of risk
Need for confirmation if risk is high

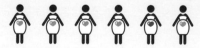

DIAGNOSIS
Invasive techniques (amniocentesis, choriocentesis)
Expensive techniques
Definitive response (yes or no)
Risk of pregnancy loss (1%)

FIGURE 51

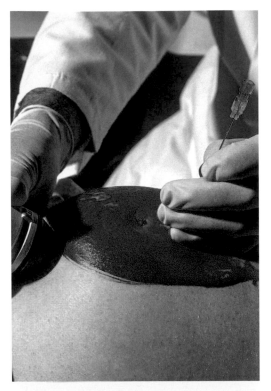

these various measurements, 96 percent of trisomy 21 cases can be detected, with only 2.5 percent of women being advised to further undergo prenatal diagnostic testing.

Most trisomies can, therefore, now be detected by the eleventh week of pregnancy, in one visit, by combining maternal characteristics, ultrasound measurements, and biochemistry of the mother's blood. But prenatal screening should no longer stop there: an in-depth assessment of the pregnancy between the eleventh and fourteenth weeks makes it possible to spot structural fetal abnormalities, as well as to predict a broad spectrum of obstetrical complications such as miscarriage, in utero fetal death, premature labour, preeclampsia, gestational diabetes, intrauterine fetal growth restriction, and fetal macrosomia.

Amniocentesis

Amniocentesis is a technique originally developed around 1880 to correct polyhydramnios, a condition in which pregnant women accumulate too much amniotic fluid. It was only after the exact number of human chromosomes had been identified and a specific chromosomal abnormality (an extra 21st chromosome) had been linked with Down syndrome that it began to be used in prenatal diagnosis toward the end of the 1960s. The fluid (approximately 20 ml) is withdrawn in a sterile procedure and the fetal cells it contains are retrieved. They are cultured for 5 to 10 days to encourage the cells to multiply; the chromosomes can then be studied.

PROBABILITY OF GIVING BIRTH TO A CHILD WITH TRISOMY 21 AS A FUNCTION OF MATERNAL AGE

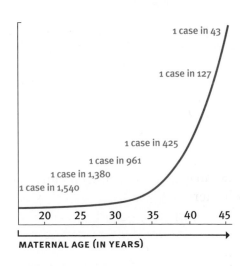

MATERNAL AGE (IN YEARS)

FIGURE 52

STRUCTURAL FETAL MALFORMATIONS

With the substantial improvement in imaging techniques, it's now possible using ultrasound between the eleventh and fourteenth weeks to detect the vast majority of serious structural (physical) malformations of the fetus, notably anencephaly, defects in the abdominal wall, spine (spina bifida) and limbs, diaphragmatic hernia, etc. More than 85 to 95 percent of heart defects are also identified early in the pregnancy through an in-depth examination of the heart, nuchal translucency, and blood flows in the ductus venosus and the tricuspid valve.

MISCARRIAGE AND INTRAUTERINE FETAL DEATH

Despite prenatal screening in the first trimester confirming the viability of the fetus, 1 percent of women will have a miscarriage between the fourteenth and twenty-first weeks and 0.4 percent will have an intrauterine fetal death after the twentieth week of pregnancy. These pregnancy complications may sometimes be detected in the first trimester by abnormally increased nuchal translucency, reversed blood flow in the ductus venosus, or an abnormally low concentration of PAPP-A in the mother's blood. While miscarriage cannot be prevented, it's quite a different story for intrauterine fetal death, which usually occurs in the third trimester of pregnancy. Patients identified during first-trimester prenatal screening as being at risk of intrauterine fetal death can benefit from closer monitoring, with increased attention paid to their wellbeing and to fetal growth. The most suitable time for delivery can thus be determined and intrauterine fetal death avoided.

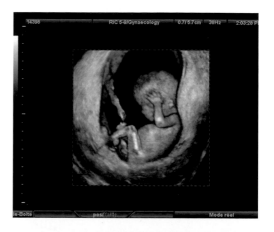

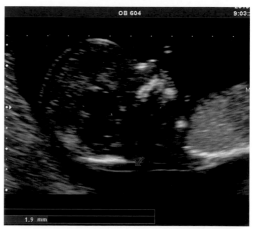

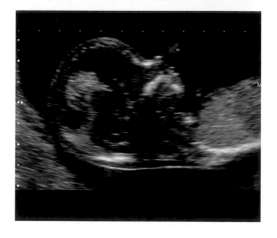

↗   Fetus in the twelfth week, visualized by 3D ultrasound.
↗   Nuchal translucency.
↗   Nasal bone.

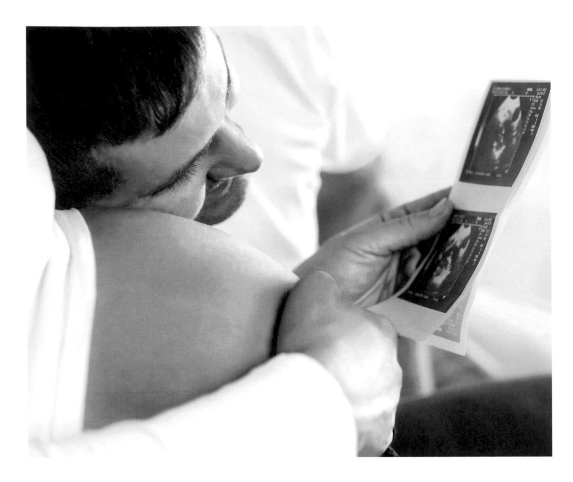

PREECLAMPSIA AND OTHER HYPERTENSIVE DISORDERS OF PREGNANCY

Formerly known as toxemia gravida, this maternal disorder is now better known by the term preeclampsia. It appears as the sudden development of high blood pressure in a woman between the twentieth week and the end of the pregnancy, accompanied by proteinuria. Preeclampsia affects from 2 to 5 percent of pregnant women and develops before the thirty-fourth week in 1 out of 250 women. If not detected in time, this disorder may result in serious complications, with the risk of fetal and maternal death, and a very premature birth, if inducing labour becomes the only way to treat it. Early screening for this condition is, therefore, very useful, especially since it has been shown that the development of the disorder can be prevented or delayed by administering low-dose aspirin to patients at risk, before the sixteenth week of pregnancy, ideally beginning in the twelfth week. Nearly 85 to 95 percent of preeclampsias that develop before the thirty-fourth week can thus be detected by means of prenatal screening in the first trimester, between the eleventh and fourteenth weeks, through a combination of maternal characteristics, average arterial blood pressure, the maternal blood concentration of PAPP-A, and the pulsatility of maternal uterine arteries, captured by Doppler during the ultrasound examination.

INTRAUTERINE GROWTH RESTRICTION

Fetuses with intrauterine growth restriction (IUGR) are exposed to higher risks of morbidity and prenatal mortality. These risks can be reduced when the condition is identified early in the pregnancy, by means of prenatal screening in the first trimester. In populations identified as being at higher risk, this method ensures increased antenatal monitoring of fetal wellbeing and growth, as well as a well-adapted and better planned delivery. To achieve this, risk prediction algorithms have been developed to detect IUGR, combining maternal characteristics, including the average arterial blood pressure, a Doppler of the uterine arteries, and the analysis of certain proteins originating from the placenta and circulating in the mother's blood. By doing prenatal screening between the eleventh and fourteenth weeks, approximately 75 percent of IUGR cases can be identified, excluding those caused by preeclampsia, detected during the same examination.

AN ARGUMENT FOR PRENATAL SCREENING IN THE FIRST TRIMESTER

Constant improvement in prenatal screening techniques makes it possible to confirm that the vast majority of malformations and phenomena leading to undesirable events develop during the first weeks of pregnancy. A high-quality prenatal screening, done early and in a single visit during the first trimester of pregnancy (between the eleventh and fourteenth weeks), means that nearly all pregnant women can now be classified as low- or high-risk for adverse events in pregnancy. Most often, they will be happily reassured.

If done properly in a clinical setting, prenatal screening in the first trimester

PYRAMID OF OBSTETRICAL VISITS (IN WEEKS)

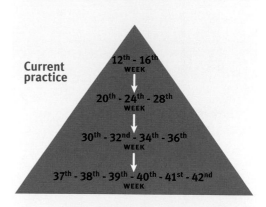

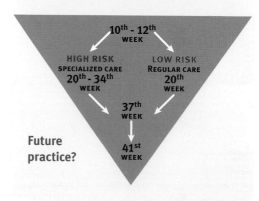

Currently, the frequency of visits increases gradually during the pregnancy, reaching its peak in the last month (upper pyramid). With prenatal screening in the first trimester, only those patients considered to be at high risk would be monitored regularly by a specialist during the first 37 weeks (lower pyramid).

FIGURE 53

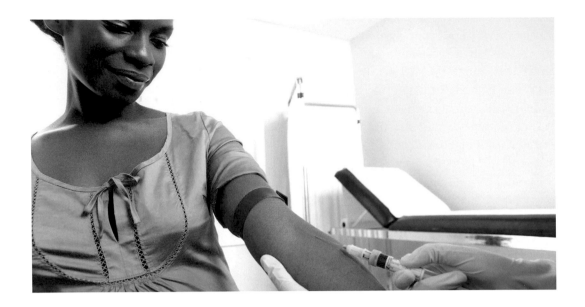

could cause a significant paradigm shift in obstetrical practice. Women identified as being at low risk of complications during pregnancy would have to undergo less medical monitoring, while those at risk would be monitored more closely by a multidisciplinary team. As a result, the pyramid of obstetrical care, as proposed by the Fetal Medicine Foundation, would be inverted (figure 53).

Other models of prenatal screening are available, including the serum integrated test in the Quebec public program. This program is very basic, as it's currently limited to screening for trisomy 21; what's more, it requires two visits (two blood tests, one between 10 and 14 weeks of pregnancy and another between 14 and 17 weeks of pregnancy). This means the result is only available very late, usually after the eighteenth week. It does not require an ultrasound in the first trimester and as a result can neither detect physical malformations of the fetus early on, nor predict undesirable events during pregnancy. We

believe, like the French and English governments, that this type of screening is out of date and does not respect basic standards of ethics and personal autonomy, even when the underlying approach is properly explained and well understood by the patient. It should be abandoned.

WHAT DOES THE FUTURE HOLD?

The fields of prenatal screening and diagnostic testing are evolving rapidly. In addition to ultrasound in the first trimester, which will certainly become more and more popular, it's likely, perhaps even inevitable, that new technologies will change our approach. As an example, tests based on the detection of fetal DNA freely circulating in maternal blood now make it possible to detect 99 percent of trisomy 21 cases and 97 percent of trisomy 18 cases using a simple maternal blood test, with no danger to the fetus. While the costs are currently exorbitant (approximately $800 CAD) and

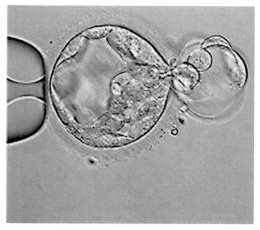

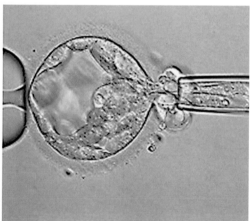

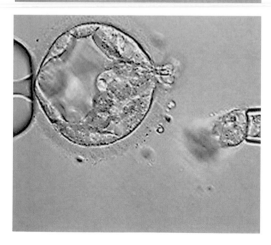

↗ Embryonic biopsy at the blastocyst stage.

these are still just screening tests (and not diagnostic tests), over time these new tests will likely become more and more affordable and be used to detect other pregnancy pathologies. In addition, research teams are actively working on tests to isolate fetal cells in the maternal bloodstream that might one day completely replace invasive methods like amniocentesis and choriocentesis. A simple maternal blood test, combined with an obstetrical ultrasound, would then be enough to arrive at a complete prenatal diagnosis.

PREIMPLANTATION SCREENING AND DIAGNOSIS

The development of diagnostic techniques could revolutionize assisted reproductive technologies. Some techniques already enable us to detect certain genetic or chromosomal abnormalities in embryos conceived through in vitro fertilization. For example, even in preliminary stages, a single cell can be retrieved from an embryo and its DNA analyzed using various molecular techniques. During screening, this kind of approach has the enormous advantage of being able to identify embryos with a chromosomal abnormality, so that only those that are healthy are selected and implanted.

During diagnostic testing, this approach is especially useful when both parents are carriers of genetic mutations that, if combined in one embryo, could cause serious diseases (cystic fibrosis, in particular). In other cases, a single mutation is enough to trigger a disease (for example, hemophilia) and analyzing products of conception means that implanting an embryo genetically predestined to develop these diseases can be avoided.

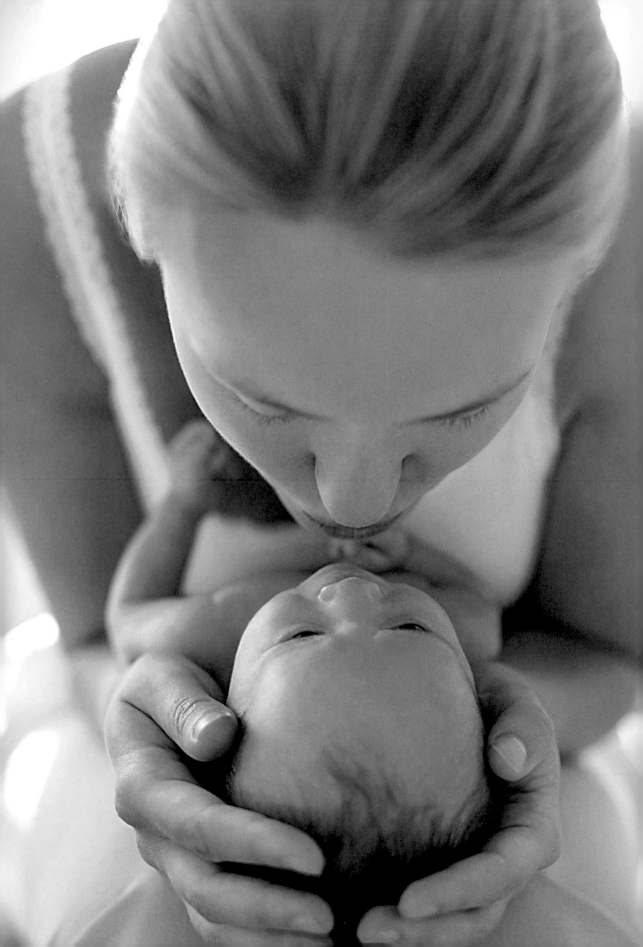

CHAPTER 8

Conceiving a Child

Every apple is a flower that has known love.
— Félix Leclerc (1914–1988)

Reproduction is such a natural process that couples who experience difficulty conceiving a child are always taken by surprise when their attempts fail repeatedly. Disappointment, sadness, anxiety, and sometimes even a feeling of unfairness over the time it's taking them to conceive can greatly disrupt these couples' lives, while leaving them confused as to the steps to take in the hope of achieving their dreams of having a child.

These feelings are completely justified, but it's important to remain positive in the face of the challenge posed by a difficulty in conceiving. There are, in fact, a number of lifestyle changes that can significantly improve fertility, and putting these preliminary steps into practice may in many cases be enough to resolve the problem. Nor must the hope of conceiving a child be abandoned even when infertility is caused by major physiological

disorders: reproductive medicine is a constantly evolving field, able to treat a significant number of hormonal and anatomical disorders, and these techniques now enable millions of people to conceive a child.

In conclusion, we would like to provide a brief overview of the main factors scientifically recognized to influence fertility, as well as the available medical procedures to overcome male and female reproductive system abnormalities.

1. MAKE LOVE OFTEN!

This may seem obvious, but it's important to remember that the frequency of sexual relations has a direct effect on the likelihood of conceiving a child. In the short term, such a "requirement" does not usually pose a problem; however, for couples who have to come to terms with repeated failures to conceive, maintaining a high level of sexual activity can become emotionally difficult in the longer term, and it's tempting to space out intercourse by "programming" it to take place at a time when success is most likely.

This kind of synchronization can, however, be harder to achieve than is generally thought. Most pregnancies are the result of intercourse that took place within a short phase of the menstrual cycle, beginning five days before ovulation and ending immediately after ovulation has occurred (figure 54). Sexual relations that occur during the last three days of this critical period (the day of ovulation and the two days beforehand) are linked to the highest probability of conception.

However, this optimal fertility window varies greatly from one cycle to another, even in women with regular cycles. A 28-day cycle, for example, does not automatically mean ovulation on day 14 and, therefore, a fertile period starting on day 9 or 10; in practice, studies show that 70 percent of women can be fertile before day 10 and after day 17 of the cycle. As a result, it's usually hard to guess the exact time of optimal fertility and limit intercourse to this period, especially when cycles are irregular. Obviously, regular menstrual cycles longer than 35 days usually require medical consultation right from the start.

Although daily sex is, in theory, associated with a greater likelihood of conception, it's generally thought that frequent sexual relations, every two or three days, is the most realistic way to maximize the chances of conception. At that rate, there remain enough sperm in the semen and they can survive up to five days in the female reproductive tract, which increases their likelihood of being close to the egg when it's released from the ovary.

PROBABILITY OF CONCEPTION ACCORDING TO THE DAY OF THE MENSTRUAL CYCLE

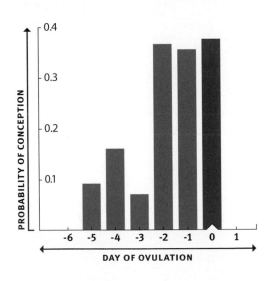

FIGURE 54 Source: Adapted from Wilcox et al., 1995.

2. IF POSSIBLE, DON'T WAIT UNTIL THE LAST MINUTE!

Family planning has enabled many women to harmoniously integrate the arrival of children into their lives, without compromising their personal and professional aspirations. The power to choose the moment to start a family is not, however, absolute: fertility decreases significantly with age and this decline alone is responsible for a large proportion of long time frames for conception. Life is unpredictable and it's impossible to completely control all of the

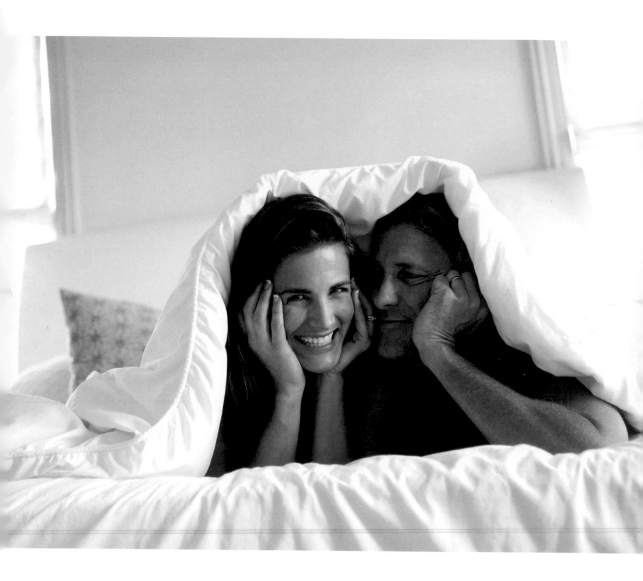

events that occur, but, when conditions permit, women who want children would be well advised not to wait too long before beginning to try to conceive, ideally before age thirty-five.

Age does not have the same effect on male fertility, but recent studies have reported a decline in the quality of sperm with age. This deterioration, which especially affects the DNA structure in the head of sperm cells, may dramatically increase the risk of certain abnormalities, like schizophrenia and autism spectrum disorder. Men who meet their partner later in life will, in the vast majority of cases, have completely normal children; they would, nonetheless, be wise to be especially vigilant and adopt the healthiest lifestyle they can (healthy diet, regular exercise, no smoking) to minimize toxic attacks on the stem cells that produce sperm and thus reduce the risk of damaging their genetic material and transmitting diseases to the child.

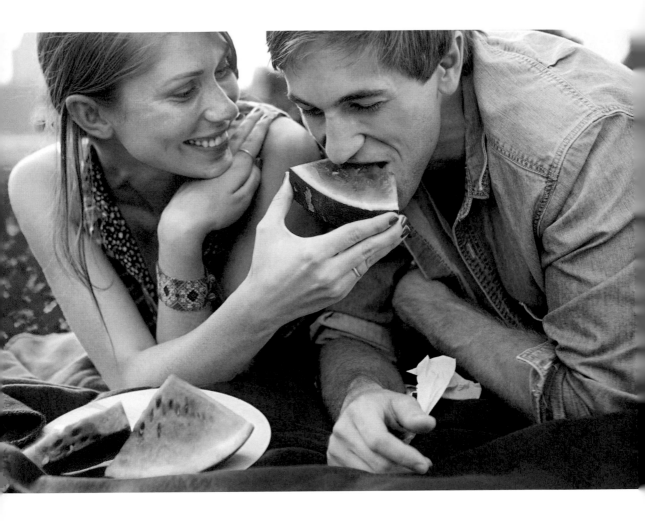

3. PUT OUT THAT CIGARETTE!

Cigarette smoking is still the principal risk factor for premature death, mainly because of the staggering increase in the risk of lung cancer and heart and lung disease that stems directly from smoking. In addition to these catastrophic effects on health, the four thousand or so chemical substances in cigarette smoke also have a number of negative effects on all reproductive functions, in women and men alike. Whether because of abnormalities in the maturation of follicles during the ovulatory cycle, a decline in the receptiveness of the uterus to the embryo or a significant increase in the risk of ectopic pregnancy, women who smoke are much more likely to experience problems conceiving, both during natural cycles and while undergoing assisted reproductive technologies procedures. Women who smoke are roughly 50 percent less likely to conceive than women who don't. In men, smoking reduces sperm production and creates oxidative stress that damages their DNA and thus makes them less able to fertilize an egg. And the enormous cancer-causing potential of tobacco smoke must not be underestimated: people who smoke a pack of cigarettes daily are estimated to accumulate approximately six hundred mutations in the genetic material in their lungs every year, and it's a certainty that some of these mutations also affect the DNA in reproductive cells and can be passed on to a child. All of these factors make quitting smoking the lifestyle change that can have the greatest positive impact on fertility ... and overall health.

4. EAT BETTER!

It's often said: "You are what you eat," and this saying is especially true where fertility is concerned. Like all cells in the body, the functioning of female and male reproductive cells is strongly influenced by conditions within the organism, and it's important to be careful to avoid metabolic imbalances that may disrupt the integrity and the maturation of these cells. In many ways, the best diet for maximum fertility is the same one recommended for the prevention of all chronic diseases (heart disease, Type 2 diabetes, and several kinds of cancer) (figure 55).

Choose Your Fats Carefully
Several studies indicate that the kinds of fats in the diet influence fertility. In this regard, the monounsaturated/trans fat relationship seems to be especially important, and this ratio can be optimized by choosing to consume sources of monounsaturated fats (olive oil, nuts, some fruits like avocado), while avoiding processed foods containing partially hydrogenated oils (fried foods, junk food in general) as much

as possible. Since the modern diet is also deficient in omega-3 fatty acids, increasing intake of dietary sources of these fats (flax seeds, fatty fish like salmon) will have positive consequences for fertility.

Reduce Blood Sugar Fluctuations
Consuming rapidly digestible sugars leads to significant fluctuations in insulin and blood sugar levels. When they recur regularly, these fluctuations tend to create a chronic inflammatory environment that interferes with the maturation of reproductive cells. A simple and effective way to better control blood sugar is to limit as much as possible the consumption of simple sugars and refined flours, often found in large amounts in processed foods. On the other hand, foods containing dietary fibre and complex carbohydrates, like vegetables, pulses, and whole grains, cause less insulin to be secreted and help stabilize blood sugar.

Choose a Variety of Protein Sources
It's not always necessary to eat meat to ensure an adequate protein intake. In fact, studies show that women who eat protein from vegetable sources (pulses, nuts, and grains) have a lower risk of ovulatory disorders than those who eat only red meat.

Specific Foods
Eating generous amounts of foods high in non-heme iron (tofu, beans, lentils, spinach) is associated with a reduction in ovulatory disorders. A high intake of iodine is also beneficial and can easily be met by incorporating foods from the sea (fish, seafood, algae) into the menu. Women trying to conceive are usually advised to take folic acid supplements, but that does not mean they have to ignore

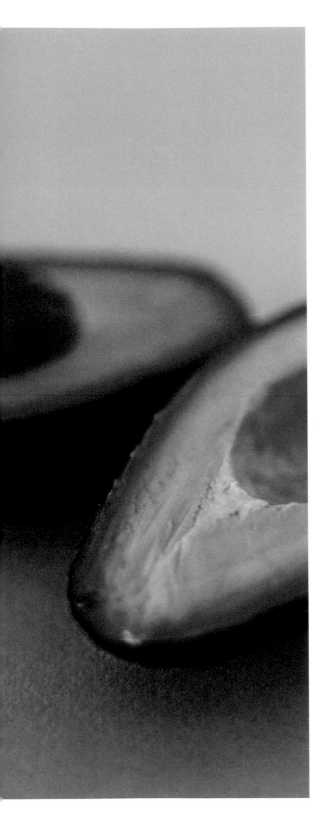

natural sources of this vitamin, such as green vegetables, high in many vitamins and minerals essential for health.

5. WATCH YOUR WEIGHT!

Once relatively rare, being overweight and obesity now affect two-thirds of the inhabitants of western countries and are currently the main risk factors for chronic disease. In terms of fertility, this extra weight can also have serious consequences, since it's clearly established that women with a body mass index higher than 25 have a greater risk of conception problems, especially when they become obese (BMI > 30) (figure 56). In men, being overweight or obese is also linked to infertility, including a greater prevalence of oligozoospermia and azoospermia (figure 57).

Maintaining a healthy weight is a difficult goal to reach for many people, not only due to the abundance of food all around us, but also because of the low energy expenditure required to carry out our daily activities. To avoid these "traps" of modern life, the best solution is still to take a defensive position against processed foods overloaded with sugar and bad fats (and thus calories) and to redefine the way we eat, by choosing, for example, a diet based on the foods described in the preceding section. Combined with moderate but regular physical activity (thirty minutes of walking daily, for example), changing these habits makes it possible to avoid having to deal with blood sugar problems, while allowing the internal mechanisms involved in appetite control to function at their best and thus avoid caloric overload.

MAIN FOODS THAT CAN INFLUENCE FERTILITY*

FOODS TO CHOOSE	FOODS TO EAT IN MODERATION
FRUITS AND VEGETABLES	
Vegetables high in folate (spinach, watercress, etc.).	Very sugary processed fruit juice.
Plants high in unsaturated fats (avocado, nuts, flax seeds, etc.).	
Vegetables and fruits high in antioxidants: red beets, prickly pears, capers, hot pepper, red onion (raw), broccoli, currants, apples, blueberries, cherries.	
MEATS AND OTHER SOURCES OF PROTEIN	
Plant proteins (pulses, nuts, grains).	Very fatty meats.
Iron-rich foods (tofu, lentils, beans).	Deli meats.
Fish, including those high in omega-3.	
Poultry.	
Lean red meat.	
STARCHES	
Whole grains.	White bread, white rice, mashed potatoes, etc.
Breads and pasta made from whole grains.	
Brown rice.	
DESSERTS	
Dark chocolate (20 g per day).	Pastries high in trans or saturated fats.
Fruits.	
Yogurt, ice cream.	Cakes, cookies made with white flour.
BEVERAGES	
Milk (3.25 %).	Coffee (<2 per day).
Green tea.	Alcohol (<2 drinks a week).
Red wine.	Soft drinks.

* The same foods are recommended during pregnancy, except alcohol, including wine, which should be prohibited.

FIGURE 55

6. ASSISTED REPRODUCTIVE TECHNOLOGY: THE MALE FACTOR

Although improving lifestyle habits can have a positive influence on fertility, several reproductive disorders are caused by serious physiological or anatomical disorders, requiring medical intervention to correct them.

When couples have failed to conceive for at least a year, one of the first steps in the investigation procedure is to determine whether this infertility could be caused by sperm abnormalities. This "male factor" may take the form of an insufficient amount of sperm (oligozoospermia or azoospermia), inadequate motility (asthenozoospermia) or morphological malformations (teratozoospermia). Most of the time, these abnormalities can be easily detected using a semen analysis. The assisted reproductive technology strategy most likely to overcome the problem can then be immediately determined (figure 58). For example, if there are serious abnormalities (absence or total immobility of sperm), more detailed analyses can determine the involvement of anatomical or hormonal factors and, eventually, make it possible to correct these problems by means of surgical interventions or drugs. When the abnormalities are less severe or the semen analysis seems normal (unexplained infertility), intrauterine insemination using concentrated preparations of sperm can be tried, but for a limited period of time. In many cases, in vitro fertilization will in the end offer the best prognosis.

RELATIVE RISK OF OVULATORY DISORDERS BY MATERNAL BODY MASS INDEX

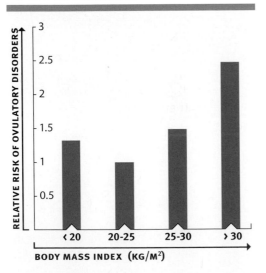

FIGURE 56   Source: Adapted from Chavarro et al., 2007.

CORRELATION BETWEEN PATERNAL BODY MASS INDEX AND PREVALENCE OF OLIGOZOOSPERMIA/AZOOSPERMIA

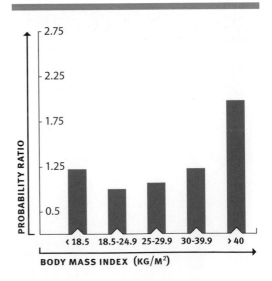

FIGURE 57   Source: Adapted from N. Sermondade et al., 2012.

EXPLORING MALE FERTILITY:
ABNORMAL SEMEN ANALYSIS

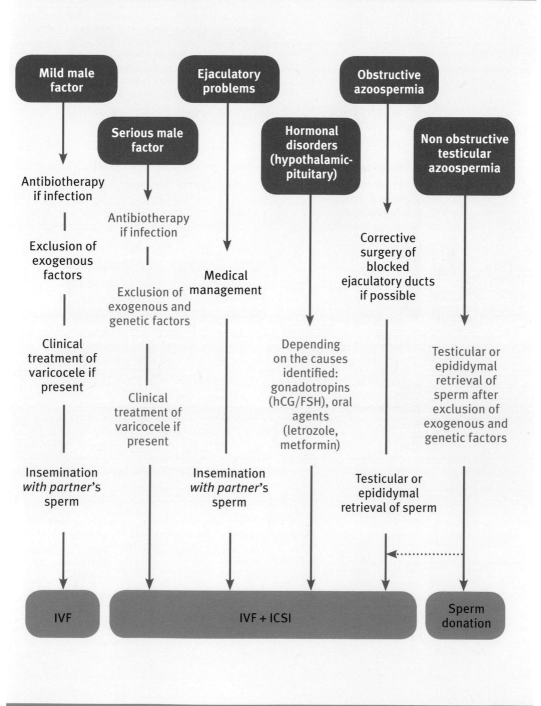

FIGURE 58

INVESTIGATING FEMALE FERTILITY

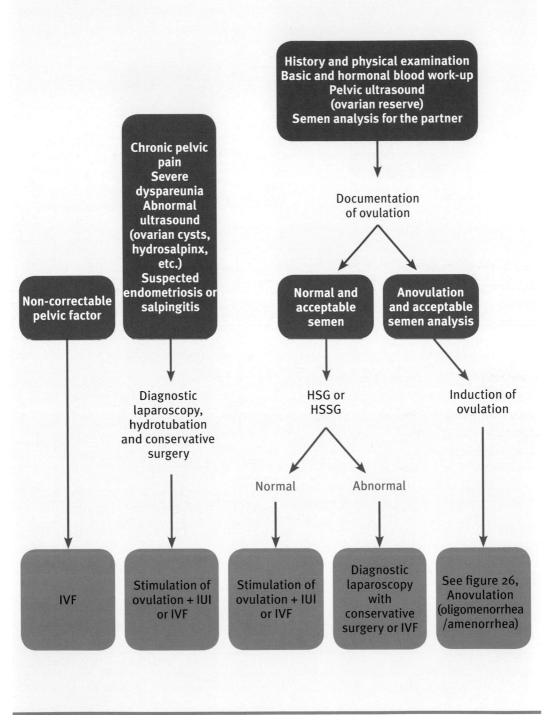

FIGURE 59

162

7. ASSISTED REPRODUCTIVE TECHNOLOGY: THE FEMALE FACTOR

A number of female fertility problems are caused by ovulatory disorders and investigation focuses on determining the causes of anovulation (figure 59). A complete hormonal profile is usually needed, so that it can be determined right away if the problem might be caused by too much prolactin in the blood or a malfunctioning thyroid gland, two conditions that can be treated quickly with drugs. In most cases, however, anovulation stems from a more subtle hormone imbalance and the goal is to determine its underlying causes. If estrogen levels are high enough to support the development of the uterine lining during the menstrual cycle, administering progestin will cause withdrawal bleeding, indicating that anovulation is caused by a hypothalamic dysfunction or polycystic ovary syndrome. Administering oral agents like clomiphene, alone or in combination with a normalization of metabolism (weight loss, metformin), can often reset ovulation and result in pregnancy. If estrogen levels are too low, the progestin will not produce withdrawal bleeding, which means that anovulation may be caused by hypothalamic-pituitary insufficiency. GnRH or gonadotropins must then be administered. Anovulation can also be due to premature disappearance of the ovarian reserve (menopause) and, in such cases, the only solution is egg or embryo donation, or adoption. In some rarer cases, usually following a curettage after a miscarriage, a delivery, or an abortion, scars (synechiae) may form in the uterine cavity and prevent the endometrium from growing in response to estrogen (Asherman's syndrome). Depending on the extent of the scarring, fertility can be restored by means of hysteroscopic surgery.

However, as with male infertility, in vitro fertilization is in many cases the only avenue possible after repeated failures with these various basic treatments.

8. PREGNANT AT LAST!

For people who've had to wait several years before succeeding in conceiving a child, a positive pregnancy test is a highly emotionally charged moment, the crowning achievement at the end of a long obstacle-filled journey. The joy this news brings must not, however, make couples forget that pregnancy is an even more important stage in the process of conception, since it has such a huge influence on the child's lifetime health.

From a dietary point of view, the main challenge for a pregnant woman is to provide the nutrients essential for fetal growth, but without subjecting the fetus to the excesses of the modern diet. It's worth repeating: you do not have to eat for two — just twice as well. The fetus's energy needs are relatively modest and easy to meet, especially in our era of overabundant food. It's mainly the quality of the modern diet that is problematic, both for what it lacks and for what it has too much of: on the one hand, too much sugar, refined flours, and bad fats that disrupt the metabolism and create blood sugar imbalances; on the other, a lack of fibre, essential polyunsaturated fats and protective antioxidants that lower our natural defences against chronic inflammation. Re-establishing the balance by avoiding processed products made with

About the Authors

DR. PIERRE MIRON, MD, PH.D., FRCSC

A specialist in reproductive medicine, Dr. Pierre Miron received his medical degree from the Université de Sherbrooke in 1980. In 1985, he obtained his degree in obstetrics and gynecology from the Université de Montréal and decided to further his studies in reproductive endocrinology and infertility at the Royal Women's Hospital at the University of Melbourne, in Australia. On his return, he founded three in vitro fertilization programs in Quebec: the Hôpital Maisonneuve-Rosemont program in Montreal (1986), PROCREA Montréal (1990), and PROCREA Québec (1998).

Dr. Miron was a professor in the Faculty of Medicine at the Université de Montréal from 1985 to 2010. He obtained a second doctorate (2011) after having founded, in 2007, the Centre de procreation Fertilys, on Montreal's north shore, now based in Laval.

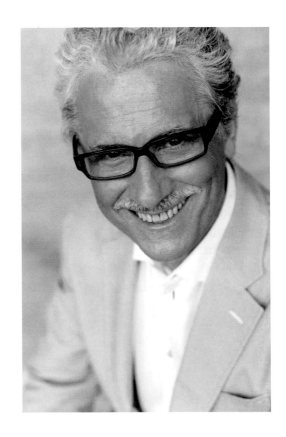

Dr. Miron has been a member of the Committee on Reproductive Endocrinology and Infertility of the Society of Obstetricians and Gynecologists of Canada (SOGC), the editorial board of the SOGC journal and the SOGC-Canadian Fertility and Andrology Society Joint Ethics Committee. For many years he chaired the Comité d'endocrinologie de la reproduction et infertilité de l'Association des obstétriciens-gynécologues du Québec (AOGQ) and sat on its board of directors. During this time he succeeded in having infertility recognized as a disease. Dr. Miron sits on the knowledge transfer committee of the Réseau Québécois en reproduction and on the prenatal screening committee of the AOGQ. Recently, he agreed to be a member of the examination board for the subspecialist program in Gynecologic Reproductive Endocrinology & Infertility of the Royal College of Physicians and Surgeons of Canada.

During his career, Dr. Miron's driving passion has been his desire to improve outcomes for infertile couples in Quebec. He participated in founding two Quebec associations for infertile couples, in addition to spending twenty-five years lobbying various government authorities, with the result that the Quebec government now covers all costs related to infertility treatments.

DR. MATHIEU PROVENÇAL, PH.D., DEPD, CSPQ

Dr. Mathieu Provençal, a clinical biochemist, obtained his doctorate in physiology from the Faculty of Medicine at the Université de Montréal in 2009. His research, carried out at the CHU Sainte-Justine in

Dr. Richard Béliveau's laboratory and published in specialized cancer journals, highlights the connection between the role of the molecules involved in activating coagulation and the development of certain types of brain cancer in children.

In 2009, Dr. Provençal began a residency in clinical biochemistry as part of a postdoctoral internship at the Université de Montréal. He obtained his postdoctoral diploma in 2011, followed by the Province of Quebec's specialist certification. Since 2011, Dr. Provençal has been working at the Hôpital Maisonneuve-Rosemont as head of the clinical endocrinology and andrology laboratories.

Appointed director of the Fertilys biomedical laboratory in 2011, he supervises its prenatal screening biochemical program.

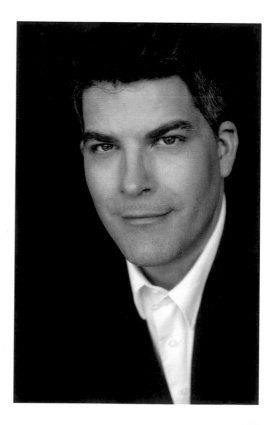

To Learn More ...

Chapter 1: The Benefits of Sex

DEY, S.K. "How We Are Born." *The Journal of Clinical Investigation* 120 (2010): 952–55.

IKAWA, M., N. INOUE, A.M. BENHAM, and M. OKABE. "Fertilization: A Sperm's Journey to and Interaction with the Oocyte." *The Journal of Clinical Investigation* 120 (2010): 984–94.

Chapter 2: Conception Difficulties

ALVAREZ, S., AND C. FALLET. "Role of Toxic Factors in the Fecundity of the Couple." *Journal de Gynécologie Obstétrique and Biologie de la Reproduction* (Paris) 39 (2010): 39–40.

ANDERSON, K., V. NISENBLAT, AND R. NORMAN. "Lifestyle Factors in People Seeking Infertility Treatment — A Review." *Australian and New Zealand Journal of Obstetrics and Gynaecology* 50 (2010): 8–20.

BRANCH, D.W., M. GIBSON, and R.M. SILVER. "Clinical Practice. Recurrent Miscarriage." *New England Journal of Medicine* 363 (2010): 1740–47.

BUSHNIK, T., J.L. COOK, A.A. YUZPE, S. TOUGH, and J. COL-LINS. "Estimating the Prevalence of Infertility in Canada." *Human Reproduction* 27 (2012): 738–46.

JOFFE, M. "What Has Happened to Human Fertility?" *Human Reproduction* 25 (2010): 295–307.

MÉNÉZO, Y., F. ENTEZAMI, I. LICHTBLAU, M. COHEN, S. BELLOC, AND M. BRACK. "Oxidative Stress and Fertility: False Evidence and Bad Recipes." *Gynécologie, obstétrique et fertilité* 40 (2012): 787–96.

WALLACE, W.H., and T. KELSEY. "Human Ovarian Reserve from Conception to the Menopause.", *PLOS ONE* 5 (2010): e8772.

WOODRUFF, T.J., S.J. JANSSEN, L.J. GUILLETTE, and L.C. GIUDICE. *Environmental Impacts on Reproductive Health and Fertility.* Cambridge: Cambridge University Press, 2010.

Chapter 3: Female Infertility

ABOULGHAR, M., and B. RIZK. *Ovarian Stimulation.* Cambridge: Cambridge University Press, 2010.

BRIOUDE, F., C.E. BOUVATTIER, and M. LOMBES. "Hypogonadotropic Hypogonadism: New Aspects in the Regulation of Hypothalamic-Pituitary-Gonadal

Axis." *Annales d'Endocrinologie* 71, suppl. 1 (2010): S33–41.

Burney, R.O., and L.C. Giudice. "Pathogenesis and Pathophysiology of Endometriosis." *Fertility and Sterility* 98 (2012): 511–19.

"Diagnostic Evaluation of the Infertile Female: A Committee Opinion." *Fertility and Sterility* 98 (2012): 302–07.

"Health and fertility in World Health Organization Group 2 Anovulatory Women." *Human Reproduction Update* 18 (2012): 586–99.

Heffner, L.J. "Advanced Maternal Age – How Old Is Too Old?" *New England Journal of Medicine* 351 (2004): 1927–29.

Jacquesson, L., J. Belaisch-Allart, and J.P. Ayel. "Induction of Ovulation." *Journal de Gynécologie Obstétrique et Biologie de la Reproduction* (Paris) 39 (2010): S67–74.

Pritts, E.A. "Letrozole for Ovulation Induction and Controlled Ovarian Hyperstimulation." *Current Opinion in Obstetrics and Gynecology* 22 (2010): 289–94.

Torre, A., and H. Fernandez. "Polycystic Ovary Syndrome (PCOS)." *Journal de Gynécologie Obstétrique et Biologie de la Reproduction* (Paris) 36 (2007): 423–46.

Chapter 4: Male Infertility

Agarwal, A., and L.H. Sekhon. "The Role of Antioxidant Therapy in the Treatment of Male Infertility." *Human Fertility* (Cambridge) 13 (2010): 217–25.

Avendano, C., A. Mata, C.A. Sanchez Sarmiento, and G.F. Doncel. "Use of Laptop Computers Connected to Internet Through Wi-Fi Decreases Human Sperm Motility and Increases Sperm DNA Fragmentation." *Fertility and Sterility* 97 (2012): 39–45 e2.

Cohen-Bacrie, P., S. Belloc, Y.J. Menezo, P. Clément, J. Hamidi, and M. Benkhalifa. "Correlation Between DNA Damage and Sperm Parameters: A Prospective Study of 1,633 Patients." *Fertility and Sterility* 91 (2009): 1801–05.

De Souza, G.L., and J. Hallak. "Anabolic Steroids and Male Infertility: A Comprehensive Review." *BJU International* 108 (2011): 1860–65.

"Diagnostic Evaluation of the Infertile Male: A Committee Opinion." *Fertility and Sterility* 98 (2012): 294–301.

Gaskins, A.J., D.S. Colaci, J. Mendiola, S.H. Swan, and J.E. Chavarro. "Dietary Patterns and Semen Quality in Young Men." *Human Reproduction* 27 (2012): 2899–907.

Gharagozloo, P., and R.J. Aitken. "The Role of Sperm Oxidative Stress in Male Infertility and the Significance of Oral Antioxidant Therapy." *Human Reproduction* 26 (2011): 1628–40.

Kim, E.D., L. Crosnoe, N. Bar-Chama, M. Khera, and L.I. Lipschultz. "The Treatment of Hypogonadism in Men of Reproductive Age." *Fertility and Sterility* 99 (2013): 718–24.

Krausz, C. "Male Infertility: Pathogenesis and Clinical Diagnosis." *Best Practice & Research: Clinical Endocrinology & Metabolism* 25 (2001): 271–85.

Morgante, G., C. Tosti, R. Orvieto, M.C. Musacchio, P. Piomboni, and V. De Leo. "Metformin Improves Semen Characteristics of Oligo-Teratoasthenozoospermic Men With Metabolic Syndrome." *Fertility and Sterility* 95 (2011): 2150–02.

Patry, G., K. Jarvi, E.D. Grober, and K.C. Lo. "Use of the Aromatase Inhibitor Letrozole to Treat Male Infertility." *Fertility and Sterility* 92 (2009): 829 e1–2.

Rolland, M., J. Le Moal, V. Wagner, D. Royère, and J. De Mouzon. "Decline in Semen Concentration and Morphology in a Sample of 26,609 Men Close to General Population Between 1989 and 2005 in France." Human Reproduction 28 (2013): 462–70.

Sakkas, D., and J.G. Alvarez. "Sperm DNA Fragmentation: Mechanisms of Origin, Impact on Reproductive Outcome, and Analysis." *Fertility and Sterility* 93 (2010): 1027–36.

SERMONDADE, N., et al. "BMI in Relation to Sperm Count: An Updated Systematic Review and Collaborative Meta-Analysis." *Human Reproduction Update* 19 (2013): 221–31.

SPANO, M., J.P. BONDE, H.I. HJOLLUND, H.A. KOLSTAD, E. CORDELLI, and G. LETER. "Sperm Chromatin Damage Impairs Human Fertility. The Danish First Pregnancy Planner Study Team." *Fertility and Sterility* 73 (2000): 43–50.

Chapter 5: Assisted Reproductive Technologies

ALI, A., M. BENKHALIFA, and P. MIRON. "In-Vitro Maturation of Oocytes: Biological Aspects." *Reproductive BioMedicine Online* 13 (2006): 437–46.

BIGGERS, J.D. "IVF and Embryo Transfer: Historical Origin and Development." *Reproductive BioMedicine Online* 25 (2012): 118–27.

CASPER, R.F., and M.F. MITWALLY. "A Historical Perspective of Aromatase Inhibitors for Ovulation Induction." *Fertility and Sterility* 98 (2012): 1352–55.

DAVIES, M.J., V.M. MOORE, K.J. WILLSON, P. VAN ESSEN, K. PRIEST, H. SCOTT, E.A. HAAN, and A. CHAN. "Reproductive Technologies and the Risk of Birth Defects." *New England Journal of Medicine* 366 (2012): 1803–13.

Fertility: Assessment and Treatment for People with Fertility Problems [Internet]. London (UK). National Institute for Health and Clinical Excellence: Guidance; RCOG Press. 2013.

GNOTH, C., B. MAXRATH, T. SKONIECZNY, K. FRIOL, E. GODEHARDT, and J. TIGGES. "Final ART Success Rates: A 10 Years Survey." *Human Reproduction* 26 (2011): 2239–46.

GRADY, R., N. ALAVI, R. VALE, M. KHANDWALA, and S. D. MCDONALD. "Elective Single Embryo Transfer and Perinatal Outcomes: A Systematic Review and Meta-Analysis." *Fertility and Sterility* 9 (2012): 324–31.

KOHLS, G., F. RUIZ, M. MARTINEZ, E. HAUZMAN, G. DE LA FUENTE, A. PELLICER, and J.A. GARCIA- VELASCO. "Early Progesterone Cessation After In Vitro Fertilization/Intracytoplasmic Sperm Injection: A Randomized, Controlled Trial." *Fertility and Sterility* 98 (2012): 858–62.

KOVACS, GAB (ed). *How to Improve Your ART Success Rates*. Cambridge: Cambridge University Press. 2011.

LAMAZOU, F., A. LEGOUEZ, V. LETOUZEY, M. GRYNBERG, X. DEFFIEUX, C, TRICHOT, H. FERNANDEZ, and R. FRYDMAN. "Ovarian Hyperstimulation Syndrome: Pathophysiology, Risk Factors, Prevention, Diagnosis and Treatment." *Journal de Gynécologie Obstétrique et Biologie de la Reproduction* (Paris) 40 (2011): 593–611.

MIRON, P., S. TALBOT, M. RIVARD, and J. LAMBERT. "Effectiveness of IVF for Unexplained Infertility and Minimal to Mild Endometriosis-Associated Infertility." *Journal of Obstetrics and Gynaecology Canada* 23 (2001): 127–31.

MORAGIANNI, V.A., S.M. JONES, and D.A. RYLEY. "The Effect of Body Mass Index on the Outcomes of First Assisted Reproductive Technology Cycles." *Fertility and Sterility* 98 (2012): 102–08.

NYGREN, K.G. "Single Embryo Transfer: The Role of Natural Cycle/Minimal Stimulation IVF in the Future." *Reproductive BioMedicine Online* 14 (2007): 626–27.

PAGIDAS, K., T. FALCONE, R. HEMMINGS, and P. MIRON. "Comparison of Reoperation for Moderate (Stage III) and Severe (Stage IV) Endometriosis-Related Infertility With In Vitro Fertilization-Embryo Transfer." *Fertility and Sterility* 65 (1996): 791–95.

PALERMO, G.D., Q.V. NERI, D. MONAHAN, J. KOCENT, and Z. ROSENWAKS. "Development and Current Applications of Assisted Fertilization." *Fertility and Sterility* 97 (2012): 248–59.

PANDEY, S., A. SHETTY, M. HAMILTON, S. BHATTACHARYA, and A. MAHESHWARI. "Obstetric and Perinatal Outcomes in Singleton Pregnancies Resulting from IVF/ICSI: A Systematic Review and Meta-Analysis." *Human Reproduction Update* 18 (2012): 485–503.

PINHEIRO, R.C., J. LAMBERT, F. BÉNARD, F. MAUFFETTE,

and P. MIRON. "Effectiveness of In Vitro Fertilization with Intracytoplasmic Sperm Injection for Severe Male Infertility." *Canadian Medical Association Journal* 161 (1999): 1397–401.

SAID, T.M., and J.A. LAND. "Effects of Advanced Selection Methods on Sperm Quality and ART Outcome: A Systematic Review." *Human Reproduction Update* 17 (2011): 719–33.

SIRISTATIDIS, C.S., S.R. DODD, and A.J. DRAKELEY. "Aspirin Is Not Recommended for Women Undergoing IVF." *Human Reproduction Update* 18 (2012): 233.

SULLIVAN, E.A., Y.A. WANG, I. HAYWARD, G.M. CHAMBERS, P. ILLINGWORTH, J. MCBAIN, and R.J. NORMAN. "Single Embryo Transfer Reduces the Risk of Perinatal Mortality, A Population Study." *Human Reproduction* 27 (2012): 3609–15.

TIITINEN, A. "Prevention of Multiple Pregnancies in Infertility Treatment." *Best Practice & Research: Clinical Obstetrics & Gynaecology* 26 (2012): 829–40.

VAN STEIRTEGHEM, A. "Celebrating ICSI's Twentieth Anniversary and the Birth of More Than 2.5 Million Children – The How, Why, When and Where." *Human Reproduction* 27 (2012): 1–2.

VERBERG, M.F., N.S. MACKLON, G. NARGUND, R. FRYDMAN, P. DEVROEY, F.J. BROEKMANS, and B.C. FAUSER. "Mild Ovarian Stimulation for IVF." *Human Reproduction Update* 15 (2009): 13–29.

Chapter 6: A Legacy of Health

BROWN, L.S., J. SHARLIN, and S. EDELSTEIN. "Nutrition Requirements During Pregnancy." In *Essentials of Life Cycle Nutrition*. Sudbury, MA (2010): Jones and Bartlett Publishers.

CALKINS, K., and S.U. DEVASKAR. "Fetal Origins of Adult Disease." *Current Problems in Pediatric and Adolescent Health Care* 41 (2011): 158–76.

EVANS, J.A. "Pre-Conceptional Vitamin/Folic Acid Supplementation" (2007). *Journal of Obstetrics and Gynaecology Canada* 30 (2008): 656–57; author's reply: 658.

GANU, R.S., R.A. HARRIS, K. COLLINS, and K.M.

AAGAARD. "Maternal Diet: A Modulator for Epigenomic Regulation During Development in Nonhuman Primates and Humans." *International Journal of Obesity Supplements* 2 (2012): S14–S18.

HOGG, K., E.M. PRICE, C.W. HANNA, and W.P. ROBINSON. "Prenatal and Perinatal Environmental Influences on the Human Fetal and Placental Epigenome." *Clinical Pharmacology and Therapeutics* 92 (2012): 716–26.

SILVEIRA, P.P., A.K. PORTELLA, M.Z. GOLDANI, and M.A. BARBIERI. "Developmental Origins of Health and Disease (DOHaD)." *Jornal de Pediatra* (Rio de Janeiro) 83 (2007): 494–504.

Chapter 7: Screening and Prenatal Diagnosis

BENN, P., H. CUCKLE, and E. PERGAMENT. "Non-Invasive Prenatal Diagnosis for Down Syndrome: The Paradigm Will Shift, But Slowly." *Ultrasound in Obstetrics & Gynecology* 39 (2012): 127–30.

BORRELL, A., M. GRANDE, M. BENNASAR, V. BOROBIO, J.M. JIMENEZ, I. STERGIOTOU, and H. CUCKLE. "First Trimester Detection of Cardiac Defects with the Use of Ductus Venosus Blood Flow." *Ultrasound in Obstetrics & Gynecology*, doi (2012): 10.1002/uog.12349.

BREZINA, P.R., D.S. BREZINA, and W.G. KEARNS. "Preimplantation Genetic Testing." *British Medical Journal* 345 (2012): e5908.

CHOOLANI, M., A.P. MAYHUDDIN, and S. HAHN. "The Promise of Fetal Cells in Maternal Blood." *Best Practice & Research: Clinical Obstetrics & Gynaecology* 26 (2012): 655–67.

CUCKLE, H. S. "Screening for Pre-Eclampsia — Lessons from Aneuploidy Screening." *Placenta* 32 Suppl (2011): S42–48.

KAGAN, K.O., I. STABOULIDOU, J. CRUZ, D. WRIGHT, and K. H. NICOLAIDES. "Two-Stage First-Trimester Screening for Trisomy 21 By Ultrasound Assessment and Biochemical Testing." *Ultrasound in Obstetrics & Gynecology* 36 (2010): 542–47.

MIRON, P., Y.P. CÔTÉ, and J. LAMBERT. "Nuchal Translucency Thresholds in Prenatal Screening for Down Syndrome and Trisomy 18." *Journal of*

Obstetrics and Gynaecology Canada 31 (2009): 227–35.

NICOLAIDES, K.H. "A Model for a New Pyramid of Prenatal Care Based on the 11 to 13 Weeks' Assessment." *Prenatal Diagnosis* 31 (2011): 3–6.

SCHOOLCRAFT, W.B., E. FRAGOULI, J. STEVENS, S. MUNNÉ, M.G. KATZ-JAFFE, and D. WELLS. "Clinical Application of Comprehensive Chromosomal Screening at the Blastocyst Stage." *Fertility and Sterility* 94 (2010): 1700–06.

SIMON-BOUY, B., D. ROYÈRE, and P. LEVY. "Sounding Board. First Trimester Down Syndrome Screening in France." *La Revue du Praticien* 62 (2012): 1340–04.

Chapter 8: Conceiving a Child

Age and Fertility: A Guide for Patients. American Society for Reproductive Medicine. 2012.

CHAVARRO, J.E., J.W. RICH-EDWARDS, B.A. ROSNER, and W.C. WILLETT. "Diet and Lifestyle in the Prevention of Ovulatory Disorder Infertility." *Obstetrics & Gynecology* 110 (2007): 1050–58.

GROLL, J., and L. GROLL. *Fertility Foods: Optimize Ovulation and Conception Through Food Choices.* New York: Fireside (Simon & Schuster). 2006.

HACKSHAW, A., C. RODECK, and S. BONIFACE. "Maternal Smoking in Pregnancy and Birth Defects: A Systematic Review Based on 173,687 Malformed Cases and 11.7 Million Controls." *Human Reproduction Update* 17 (2011): 589–604.

WILCOX, A.J., D. DUNSON, and D.D. BAIRD. "The Timing of the 'Fertile Window' in the Menstrual Cycle: Day Specific Estimates from a Prospective Study." *British Medical Journal* 321 (2000): 1259–62.

WILCOX, A.J., C.R. WEINBERG, and D.D. BAIRD. "Timing of Sexual Intercourse in Relation to Ovulation. Effects on the Probability of Conception, Survival of the Pregnancy, and Sex of the Baby." *New England Journal of Medicine* 333 (1995): 1517–21.

COORDINATES

DR. PIERRE MIRON
DR. MATHIEU PROVENÇAL

FERTILYS

1950, rue Maurice-Gauvin
Suite 103
Laval (Quebec) Canada
H7S 1Z5
Tel: (450) 934-9146
Fax: (450) 934-9156

info@fertilys.org
www.fertilys.org

ILLUSTRATION CREDITS

123RF.COM, photo_16083541: 26

CATHERINE CLARK, Fertilys: 86 (normal concentration of sperm and oligozoospermia, two images)

DR. ELISABETH LEDOUX, radiology department, CHRDL: 79 (normal and abnormal hysterosalpingograms, two images)

DR. GIOVANNA TOMASI/CRA Centro Riproduzione Assistita (Catania, Italy): 100, 107, 1st image (unfertilized egg)

DR. PIERRE MIRON: 68 (PCOS ovary), 78 (uterus and its appendages, two images), 147 (three ultrasounds)

DR. SANTIAGO MUNNÉ, Reprogenetics and Fertility and Sterility (Elsevier B.V., 2010): 151 (embryonic biopsy at the blastocyst stage, three images)

GE: 67 (3D ovarian follicles)

GETTY IMAGES: Betty Wiley/Flickr Open/Getty Images 14; Laurence Monneret/Image Bank/Getty Images 18; Tyler Stableford/Lifesize/Getty Images 21; Paul Bradbury/Riser/OJO Images/Getty Images 27; Ariel Skelley/Blend Images/Getty Images 32; Fredrik Nyman/Johner Images/Getty Images 33; DAVID M PHILLIPS/Photo Researchers/Getty Images 35; Lillian Elaine Wilson/The Image Bank/Getty Images 39; Dennis Hallinan/Archive Photos/Getty Images 40; Imagno/Hulton Archive/Getty Images 42; Philip Lee Harvey/Stone+/Getty Images 47; Zero Creatives/Cultura/Getty Images 48; Yellowdog Productions/Lifesize/Getty Images 49; FotografiaBasica/E+/Getty Images 52; Bruce Dale/National Geographic/Getty Images 54; Frank Herholdt/Stockbyte/Getty Images 55; dardespot/E+/Getty Images 56; Danielle D. Hughson/Flickr Select/Getty Images 58; Trevor Williams/Fiz-iks /Flickr/Getty Images 59; momentimages/Tetra images/Getty Images 60; ZenShui/

Frederic Cirou/PhotoAlto Agency RF Collections/Getty Images 62; James Darell/Riser/Getty Images 65; Troels Graugaard/E+/Getty Images 66; Ruth Jenkinson/Dorling Kindersley/Getty Images 69; MAURO FERMARIELLO/Science Photo Library/Getty Images 74; Graham Monro/gm photographics/Photolibrary/Getty Images 77; Peter Stackpole/Time & Life Pictures/Getty Images 82; Tatyana Aleksieva Photography/Flickr/Getty Images 85; NYPL/Science Source/Photo Researchers/Getty Images 88; BIOPHOTO ASSOCIATES/Photo Researchers/Getty Images 89; IAN HOOTON/SPL/Science Photo Library/Getty Images 91; Vladimir Piskunov/Vetta /Getty Images 96; John Lamb/Taxi/Getty Images 102; Keystone-France/Gamma-Keystone/Getty Images 105; Popperfoto/Getty Images 112; Ulrich Baumgarten/Getty Images 114; Marion C. Haßold/Flickr/Getty Images 116; Amanda Rohde/E+/Getty Images 118; Steve Allen/Stone/Getty Images 122; JGI/Blend Images/Getty Images 126; Camille Tokerud/The Image Bank/Getty Images 127; Sam Edwards/OJO Images/Getty Images 128; Gary Buss/Taxi/Getty Images 129; Shmuel Mikel Bowles/E+/Getty Images 130; Antonio M. Rosario/Photographer's Choice/Getty Images 131; Lucy Lambrieux/Flickr/Getty Images 133; Roz Woodward/Lifesize/Getty Images 134; B2M Productions/Photographer's Choice RF/Getty Images 138; Frank Herholdt/The Image Bank/Getty Images 140; DEA/G. DAGLI ORTI/De Agostini Picture Library/Getty Images 143; Will & Deni MCIntyre/Photo Researchers/Getty Images 146; dexter_s/E+/Getty Images 148; ADAM GAULT/SPL/Science Photo Library/Getty Images 150; Tom Merton/Caiaimage/Getty Images 152; Digital Vision/Getty Images 155; Image Source/Getty Images 156; Jeanene Scott/The Image Bank/Getty Images 158

YANNICK FERREIRA, Fertilys: 107, images 2 to 5 (embryos, blastocysts and morula), 110 (ICSI, one image)

MICHEL ROULEAU: 20, 22, 28, 30, 34, 36, 37, 53, 95, 98, 120, 123, 124, 135

SARAH SCOTT: 167

Coming Soon in the Your Health Series

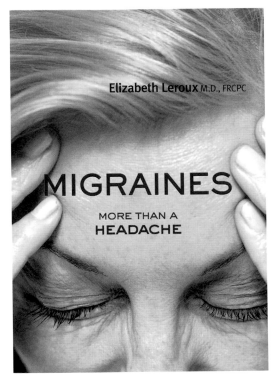

MIGRAINES
More Than a Headache
Elizabeth Leroux M.D., FRCPC

Though often viewed as a "woman's ailment," migraines affect nearly 15 percent of the world's population. In addition to the effect migraines have on the quality of life of sufferers, there is also an economic cost, caused especially by work absenteeism. But by recognizing the problem and taking necessary action, migraine sufferers today can take back control of their lives.

Written in an easy-to-read style, this comprehensive guide to migraine management answers the questions that people most often ask. The author, clinical neurologist Dr. Elizabeth Leroux, explains predispositions, triggers, and phases of migraines, as well as the three recommended lines of treatment: lifestyle changes, crisis management, and preventative therapy. Stressing the need for doctor-patient communication, this book is as much a tool for health care professionals as it is for migraine sufferers and their families.

Available at your favourite bookseller

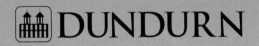
DUNDURN

VISIT US AT
Dundurn.com
@dundurnpress
Facebook.com/dundurnpress
Pinterest.com/dundurnpress